MORBID OBESITY:

THE REAL SKINNY

BY

NICK NICHOLSON M.D.

AND

B.A. BLACKWOOD

Published by Bariatric Resources Publishing
A subsidiary of Bariatric Resources, LLC

***

PUBLISHER'S NOTE

This is a compilation of observations and conclusions made and drawn during many years of treating and performing surgery upon bariatric patients by Nick Nicholson, M.D. It does not, and does not purport to, give medical advice to the reader, although hopefully it will be useful to those contemplating the use of bariatric surgery to lose weight.

ISBN: 0990436705
ISBN 13: 9780990436706

Library of Congress Control Number: 2014912337
Obesity Resources Publishing
Dallas, Texas

Acknowledgements

The publication of this book would not have been possible without the generosity and support of Northstar Healthcare Surgery Center Dallas to whom I express my most sincere thanks.

Nick Nicholson, M.D.

Table of Contents

CHAPTER ONE

Declaring War Against the Real Enemy

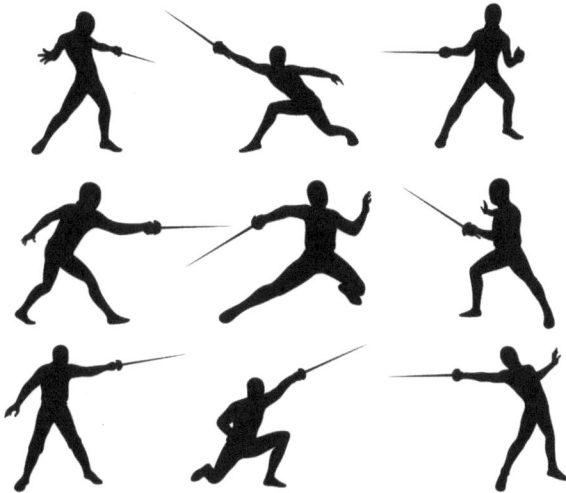

Morbid obesity is now classified as a disease, but millions of people walk around with it and seem okay. It's not ideal, but it's not like having something as scary as cancer, right?

Wrong.

Morbid obesity kills more people than cancer. In fact, the word "morbid" comes from the word "mori" meaning "to die", which is appropriate because it's directly responsible for a variety of devastating diseases.

Yet morbid obesity isn't understood or treated as something as menacing as cancer. Despite the "let's move" campaigns, the attempts to ban sugary drinks, laws requiring restaurants to cough up the calorie counts for their fried blooming onion rings and the barrage of media attention, morbid obesity is still the only lethal disease that many people choose not to treat, either through ignorance, improper medical advice, or hopelessness.

Compare the difference in a diagnosis of cancer versus one of morbid obesity. If you're unfortunate enough to receive a cancer diagnosis, you won't walk out of your doctor's office without the rudiments of a game plan which will be revisited and revised over time.

Testing, second opinions, chemotherapy, radiation, surgery – all these options will be explored, choices will be made, timelines will be considered, percentages of success for various treatments will be calculated, family members will be consulted, and, if necessary, advanced life directives signed. Patients subject themselves to whatever treatment options are available, including experimental ones if necessary.

In other words, an army of medical professionals and family enter the field ready to do battle with the cancer to the death – either of the disease or of the patient.

On the other hand, patients receiving a diagnosis of morbid obesity are usually shoved onto the battle field alone, unarmed and unprepared, equipped only with a vague admonition from their doctor to "lose weight". They have no idea of their prognosis, what their next step should be, or what treatment options have the best chance of success.

They leave their doctor's office with no game plan and no concept of how to defeat the disease.

Instead, as the years pass, their lives become all about treating the symptoms of their morbid obesity rather than the disease itself. They start taking medication for their Type II diabetes, their high blood pressure, their acid reflux, their aching joints, and their congestive heart failure. Their schedules fill up with doctor's appointments and their monthly budget for medication keeps growing.

Treating all of these diseases rather than attacking their underlying cause is like putting a pressure bandage on a gushing femoral artery. It may slow the flow of blood for a while, but it won't fix the problem. The patient will ultimately bleed out.

They're fighting a war they can't win instead of declaring war on the real culprit – morbid obesity.

And that's a tragedy, because unlike cancer, morbid obesity is one hundred percent curable. In fact, curing it and keeping it from recurring are totally within your control.

For those who have been battling their weight for years without success, the words "totally in your control" sound preposterous. After all, it's not as though you woke up one morning and decided "you know, I think I'd like to be morbidly obese" and then set about getting there. You got there over time, and for most people with the disease, you've been unable to shed the weight no matter what program you've tried. Nothing in your life has ever felt more out of control than your weight.

But you're wrong. Armed with the proper knowledge, tools and desire, you can cure your morbid obesity and keep it cured for the rest of your life. And that's the best way you can treat all the other diseases spawned by morbid obesity.

That's what this book is about – what the diagnosis means, treatment options, and long term outcomes. By the time you turn the final page, you'll know the facts you need to know about how morbid obesity impacts your life, what diseases it causes, effective treatments and how to keep it from recurring.

You'll be fighting the real enemy armed with a battle plan that will work.

CHAPTER TWO

Knowing the Enemy: What the Diagnosis Means

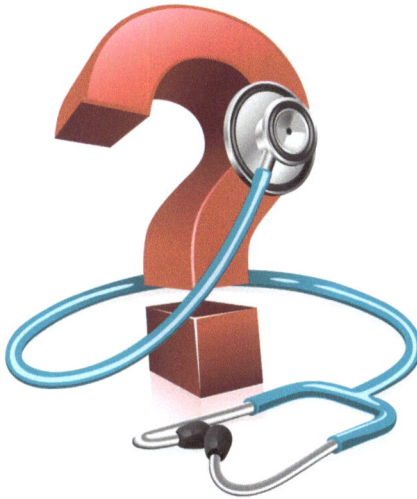

If you decide to do battle with your morbid obesity, you need to go in armed with as much knowledge as possible. Your enemy isn't going to surrender without a fight.

So let's start with the basics. You're morbidly obese if:

- You're 100 pounds or more above your ideal body weight; or

- You have a body mass index (obtained by dividing your weight in kilograms by your height squared) of 35 or over;[1] or

- You have a body mass index of 30 or over and are suffering from at least one serious obesity-related health condition.

Before you received the diagnosis or calculated your BMI, you probably had a good idea that you were morbidly obese and knew you should lose weight. What you may not know is that the diagnosis is just the tip of the iceberg.

Morbid obesity causes other deadly diseases. The odds that you'll get one or more of them isn't theoretical or limited to a small percentage of morbidly obese people. It's totally predictable and highly probable.

Obesity affects your body at a cellular level, and typically morbidly obese people will not have just one related disease; they'll have a number of conditions that all exacerbate each other, leading to the breakdown of the body, cell by cell, joint by joint, organ by organ. Most doctors treat the symptoms at an increasingly breakneck rate as the patient ages, but never effectively treat the underlying cause.

Think of morbid obesity as oxygen and the diseases it causes as fire. You can feed a fire by adding oxygen, or you can smother it by taking oxygen away. Morbid obesity acts as

---

1 If you're not a metric whiz, check out the BMI calculator at http://www.mayoclinic.org/bmi-calculator/itt-20084938

pure oxygen for Type II diabetes, cancer, heart disease, high blood pressure, congestive heart failure, liver disease, sleep apnea, degenerative joint disease, infertility, and depression. Deprive those diseases of the morbid obesity, and you can cure or improve some and wholly avoid others.

This chapter isn't meant to scare you, unless fear is what you need to go get help for the problem. It's written so that you can understand what will happen if you don't treat your morbid obesity as seriously as a diagnosis of cancer. After all, knowing your enemy is half the battle, and this is an enemy that you can defeat – no matter who you are, no matter how ill-equipped you feel.

So, here's what a diagnosis of morbid obesity means in a nutshell:

You'll die earlier.

The obesity epidemic is close to edging out smoking as the leading cause of preventable deaths among American adults. Morbid obesity causes over 300,000 deaths per year, three times the number of deaths from breast and colon cancer combined.

Depending on your race, sex, and age at the time you become morbidly obese, you'll lose 13% to 22% of your anticipated years left to live.

To put that in practical terms, if you're a 20 year old white male with a BMI of 45 or greater, you'll die thirteen years earlier than a 20 year old male with a normal BMI. So, instead of living to the age of 76, you'll most likely die at age 63, right when you're this close to those long awaited retirement plans and about the time your grandchildren are playing in little league games or soccer tournaments.

Some younger, naïve people blithely dismiss the notion of dying early, thinking that if they die at 63 rather than 76, they'll miss the years of painful decline that many older people suffer before they die. They've seen the hell their grandfather went through in the last five years of his life – who wants that?

In fact, they won't miss one second of pain by dying earlier. Instead, while their friends are out playing golf and traveling in their 50's, they'll be slowly declining because of a myriad of accumulating issues - diabetes, renal failure, reduced mobility due to degenerative joint disease, or damage caused by stroke or congestive heart failure.

Listed below are the major diseases produced by morbid obesity and how weight loss impacts them.

Type II diabetes

You're ten times more likely to have Type II diabetes if you're morbidly obese.

Ever hear of too much of a good thing? The disease takes something beneficial in your body – glucose to provide energy to your cells – and then messes with the insulin hormone responsible for delivering the glucose to your cells so that your cells get only a fraction of what they need and glucose builds up in your bloodstream.

What was meant to be a life sustaining nutrient now becomes a weapon, leading to tissue damage, kidney failure, blindness, heart attack, stroke, dementia, and arterial blockage in the legs which can result in amputation.

Medication helps, but can't totally undo the damage caused by the disease, and diabetics diagnosed in middle age live ten years less than their healthy peers.

Type II diabetes is one hundred percent curable with weight loss. Take away the morbid obesity, and the insulin hormone puts on its delivery cap again and distributes the proper amount of glucose to your cells.

<u>Cancer</u>

Cancer cells behave like the mutant organism in your favorite science fiction film. They're seriously warped and replicate at Mach speed. They don't die when they should and start taking over territory in your body like army ants.

Your risk of developing esophageal, pancreatic, colon, rectal, breast, kidney, endometrial, and liver cancer if you're morbidly obese increases anywhere from 4% to 40%, depending on the type of cancer.

So what is it about morbid obesity that makes you more susceptible to cancer?

A normal cell requires certain levels of pH, potassium, sodium and glucose both inside and outside its walls. Morbid obesity changes those levels, which damages the cell and impacts the amount of progesterone and estrogen produced in the body.

These hormone imbalances provide a fertile environment for cancer cells, creating the same effect as picking up an ugly, dying plant that got mistakenly dropped into the desert and giving it a big drink of water and a squirt of Miracle Gro.

Getting down to a healthy weight puts that plant back out in the desert to die.

High Blood Pressure

You're more likely to have high blood pressure if you're morbidly obese. The reasons for this susceptibility aren't completely understood, but there's an unquestionable link.

The walls of healthy arteries are flexible and elastic, but persistent high blood pressure causes them to harden, thicken and narrow. Think of a garden hose that was flexible when new, but then got brittle, stiff and kinked as it baked outside in the summers and froze in the winters.

Trying to force blood through rigid, thickened arteries makes your heart work double time, and no matter how hard it works it can't get the same amount of blood to your vital organs and brain as it could when your arteries were flexible and open. Even worse, sometimes the arteries narrow to the point that they become totally blocked.

The result? Increased risk of heart attacks, strokes, kidney failure and dementia.

Medications can control high blood pressure but they have their own consequences. They're expensive and can have side effects ranging from a chronic cough to weakness to impaired sexual function.

Losing weight completely cures high blood pressure in most patients and significantly lowers it for the rest.

Sleep Apnea

Morbid obesity leads to a higher risk for developing sleep apnea, in which you have one or more pauses in breathing or shallow breaths while you sleep. Although that description sounds benign, people die from it.

Morbidly obese people typically have low muscle tone and soft tissue around their airway. When they lie down to sleep, the muscles around the airway relax even further and the soft tissue collapses on itself, making it difficult to breathe. This means that your heart has to work harder and harder to pump enough oxygen rich blood throughout your body.

It's like having a single window air conditioning unit in a 3000 square foot house on a 95 degree day. The air conditioner can't properly cool the house and never gets a break. The heart of a person with sleep apnea never gets to rest and wears out before it should, just like the motor on a constantly running air conditioning unit.

This puts you at increased risk for high blood pressure, congestive heart failure, stroke, damage to blood vessels in the lungs and an irregular heartbeat. By losing down to a healthy weight, your heart settles into a normal workload and the risks associated with sleep apnea go away.

Congestive Heart Failure

Morbid obesity causes congestive heart failure, a condition in which the heart can't pump blood fast enough to meet the body's needs. Why? Because your heart is having to support more weight than it was designed for, like trying to power a speedboat with a couple of AA batteries.

As your heart struggles to keep up with your body's demands, it will stretch to hold more blood to pump through the body. This helps keep the blood moving, but causes the walls of your heart to stiffen and lose their elasticity.

Think of trying to squeeze your toothpaste from a hard plastic cylinder instead of a flexible tube. The same thing happens with your heart. It can't squeeze or contract as it should, so it can't pump as much blood, and, as a result, the kidneys may respond by causing the body to retain water and salt. If fluid builds up in the arms, legs, ankles, feet, lungs or other organs, the body becomes congested, i.e. congestive heart failure.

It's just as bad as it sounds. You can take medication, but as long as you're forcing the heart to do more work than it was designed for, the problem is only going to get worse, and will ultimately cause anything from surgery to death.

Losing down to a healthy weight lowers the stress on the heart to normal limits and takes you out of the cardiologist's office.

Gastroesophageal Reflux Disease (GERD)

Over 50% of morbidly obese people have GERD, which means that the sphincter that allows food into the stomach and closes to prevent it from flowing back up into your esophagus isn't working properly. It's that burning sensation you feel in your heart or throat caused by the backwash of stomach acid irritating your esophagus.

Although GERD can be caused by other things, in morbidly obese people it's most often caused by extra weight pressing on the intestines and stomach which causes the sphincter to relax, allowing stomach acid into the esophagus.

Besides the discomfort created by GERD, it can cause esophageal bleeding and ulcers. Even worse, the repeated exposure of acid to the esophagus is the number one cause of esophageal cancer.

Losing weight can completely resolve GERD, cutting your risk for esophageal cancer, bleeding and ulcers, and allowing you to forego its peripheral discomforts like having to sleep upright at night, taking expensive digestive medications, and undergoing annual endoscopies.

Degenerative Joint Disease

The joints of the human body were designed to support only a certain amount of weight, and when you're morbidly obese, you're over-taxing your joints, just like loading an elevator beyond its stated capacity.

Imagine lugging your twenty pound carry-on bag for ten gates at the airport and the relief you feel when you put it down. That's what your body is doing multiplied by three or five times or more, except it never gets to put the bag down. That extra weight inevitably leads to degeneration of your joints, which leads to pain in your back, hips, knees and ankles, ultimately resulting in arthritis or worse.

Even small walks seem like marathons, and you begin taking medication for your pain. You get MRI's and CT scans to pinpoint the problem joints, and you get steroid shots, knee replacements, and back surgery to try to provide some relief.

A stunning number of morbidly obese people take narcotics such as Vicodin or Hydrocodone for chronic pain, which causes constipation and impairs the ability to reason and drive. But the pain never gets better, or at least not for long, and living with chronic pain leads to personality changes. You're not as nice as you used to be, you don't want to interact with your kids or spouse, and you don't want to go out with your friends or they don't want to go out with you.

If you're fortunate enough to have escaped damage so far, you may prevent it altogether by losing weight. If you're already into the degenerative joint disease cycle, it will slow down the process, enable you to reduce or forego your pain medication, and may keep it from getting any worse. One thing is certain: if you continue to overtax your body with excess weight, your joints will deteriorate and you'll be launched into a vicious cycle of chronic pain.

Liver Disease

Liver disease used to be associated primarily with chronic alcoholics, but now obesity has overtaken alcohol as its leading cause. When you're obese, not only are your arms, thighs and abdomen storing excess fat, your liver is too. This causes the liver to grow and replace healthy liver cells with permanent scar tissue.

Why should you care? All of your blood passes through the liver, and its job is to clean out the toxins and break down nutrients from your food - as well as any medications you may take - into a form that your body can use or discard. In other words, it acts like the receiving and shipping department of a major corporation, and if it's not working properly, it can receive but can't process the blood properly to ship it out.

The liver's inability to do its job results in cirrhosis, liver cancer, and an increased risk of heart attack and stroke, any one of which can kill you.

Weight loss will prevent liver disease and may stop the liver from being damaged beyond repair in those who already have it.

Infertility

Morbidly obese women have a much harder time getting pregnant, either for mechanical reasons or because the hormone levels necessary for pregnancy have gone haywire due to the cellular changes caused by their obesity.

Taking the weight off can ease both of these problems, giving women new hope who've never had a fighting chance to get pregnant before.

Depression

Most people don't think about depression when counting the ways morbid obesity has altered their lives. But a high percentage of morbidly obese people are on anti-depressant or anti-anxiety medications, and over 50% have one or more of the classic signs of depression:

- Difficulty concentrating, remembering details, and making decisions

- Fatigue and decreased energy

- Feelings of guilt, worthlessness, and/or helplessness

- Feelings of hopelessness and/or pessimism

- Insomnia, early-morning wakefulness, or excessive sleeping

- Irritability, restlessness

- Loss of interest in activities or hobbies once pleasurable, including sex

- Persistent aches or pains, headaches, cramps, or digestive problems that do not ease even with treatment

- Persistent sad, anxious, or "empty" feelings

- Thoughts of suicide, suicide attempts

Why are you depressed when you're overweight? Because you're not doing the things you want to do and you're not happy with much of anything - your clothes, your body, your job and your relationships.

You're tired of poking yourself with a needle or choking down pills. You feel guilty that you can't do things with your kids because you're not able to climb the bleachers to attend their games. You can't play with your toddlers on the floor because you're afraid you can't get back up. You're treated differently at work, or you were passed over for that promotion you deserved. Your marriage has lost its intimacy or you've settled for a loveless relationship.

Depression can be resolved by curing its root cause – the morbid obesity that's permeated every aspect of your life.

You've probably noticed a common theme in the discussion of the diseases caused by morbid obesity. They all feed on each other, virtually ensuring that you won't escape with just one if you do nothing.

MORBID OBESITY

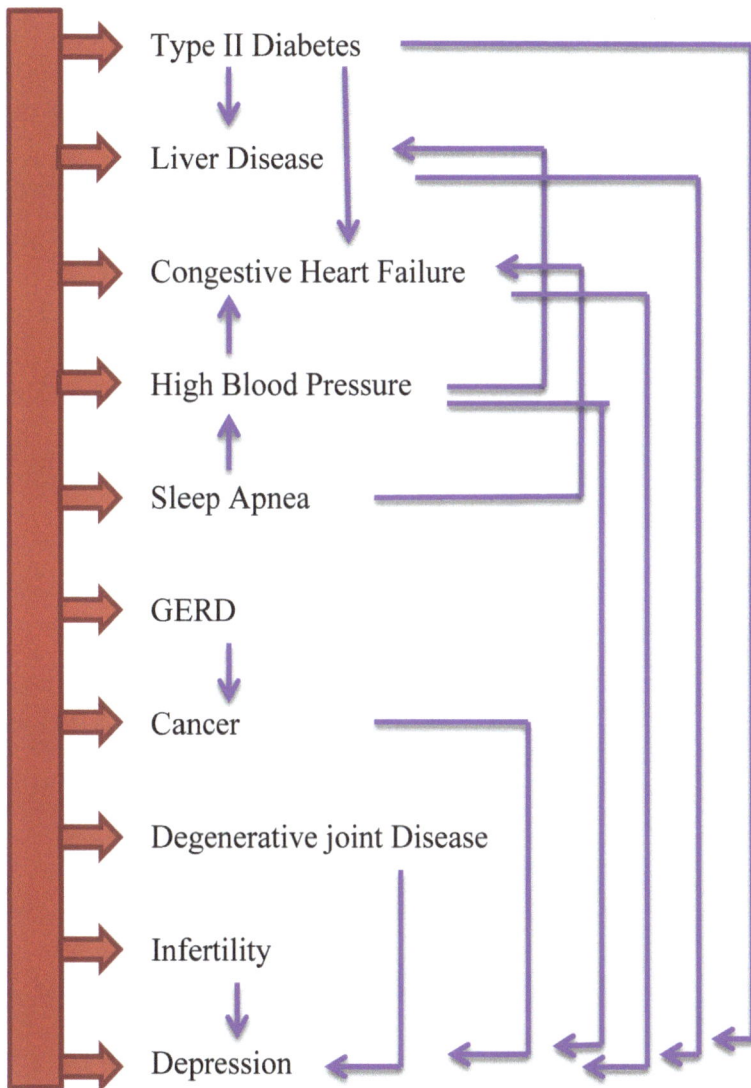

Type II Diabetes

Liver Disease

Congestive Heart Failure

High Blood Pressure

Sleep Apnea

GERD

Cancer

Degenerative joint Disease

Infertility

Depression

The bottom line: if you're morbidly obese, today is the best you're ever going to feel if you don't get down to a healthy weight.

If viewing the awful statistics gives you motivation to tackle the problem, go for it. Soon, though, as you start losing weight, you'll be motivated by optimism and not fear. The difference in your life will give you the incentive to keep going.

With the proper medical and psychological help, you can defeat this enemy.

CHAPTER THREE

Choosing a Battle Plan: Treatment Options

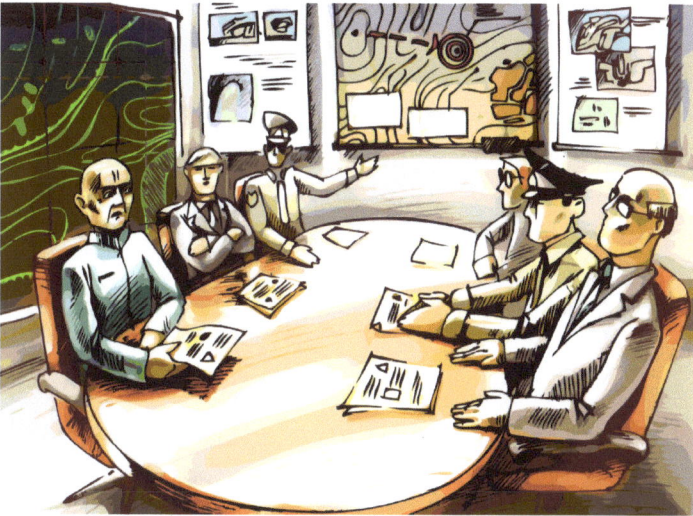

   Most diseases require you to offer up your body to treatment by others. Your job is to take the required pills or submit to surgery or endure the prescribed chemotherapy or follow the torturous exercises the physical therapist forces you through. It's scary to lose control, but there's comfort in knowing that experienced medical professionals are administering the treatment that will hopefully cure your illness.

Curing morbid obesity requires the opposite approach. Most of the treatment will be administered by you. There's no magic pill, injection or surgery that will permanently melt the pounds away. It's an active process requiring your full participation.

If you're not motivated to change your life to get healthy, no remedy in the world will work. But, your morbid obesity can absolutely be cured if you buy into the proper treatment.

Morbidly obese people have three options:

1. Do nothing;

2. Diet and exercise down to a healthy weight; or

3. Undergo weight loss surgery with its associated behavioral changes.

1. <u>Doing Nothing</u>

Most morbidly obese people would like to lose weight, but end up doing nothing by default. Some feel hopeless, believing based on past experience that no diet in the world will provide a long term solution to their problem. Others are in active denial, expending tremendous amounts of energy ignoring how they feel, look and how others treat them so they never have to face the problem.

Doing nothing may not sound like a deliberate choice, but it's like getting in your car, disabling the seatbelt, and speeding a hundred miles an hour the wrong way down a one way street.

The people ignoring the problem have turned the car stereo up full blast to drown out the warning honks and sirens following their path. The people who feel hopeless believe they have no other choice but to keep barreling along in the death car.

The result is the same. Sooner or later there will be a fiery crash and no escaping the fact that the decision to get behind the steering wheel was an active, conscious choice to cut your life short.

In other words, Option 1 guarantees you an earlier death.

2. <u>Diet and Exercise</u>

The most recommended option for morbidly obese people is diet and exercise. Sounds like the right choice – everyone knows that the key to healthy weight is diet and exercise.

So why do so many people fail at it?

If you're like most morbidly obese people, you've tried multiple diets, but losing weight and keeping it off feels harder than splitting the atom. Whether it's a physician-supervised diet or Jenny Craig or Weight Watchers or an extreme liquid diet, you've been there, done that, and gone down in flames.

You may have lost weight in the beginning, but you couldn't lose enough, and, even worse, you gained it all back and more. And exercise? You barely got down to a weight where you could walk on a treadmill without your heart racing when you started gaining the weight back.

So, you decide either that you've got the willpower of a gnat or that you just don't have the resources or time to lose weight.

The time and resources argument initially sounds good. Healthy, fresh food costs more and you're trying to feed a family of four on limited means. KFC and McDonald's fit your budget, and, besides, even if you had the money you don't have time to grocery shop and cook between your job and the kids' activities.

And exercise? Forget it. You don't have the money to join a gym or hire a personal trainer, and, even if you did, you don't have the time to work out.

The fact that puts the lie to this kind of thinking is Oprah Winfrey, someone who should be the skinniest person on the planet. She's driven, savvy, and successful. She's undeniably got will power, money and time. She has personal chefs, in-home exercise equipment, the money to buy the best food and the most motivating trainers, and the time to devote to taking care of herself. Yet she's gained, lost and regained weight just like you.

So, why don't diets work? The reason has nothing to do with your will power, your pocket book, or your busy schedule.

Here's the truth - <u>diet and exercise alone fail 98% of the time</u>.[2]

Yes, you read that right. If you're morbidly obese, you have only a 2% chance of losing down to a healthy weight and keeping it off by diet and exercise alone.

---

2   Based upon clinical studies of morbidly obese people over a 5 year period.

And it's not because morbidly obese people lack the will, character, grit, guts or determination to lose weight. It's because they're fighting an unwinnable battle with their own physiology.

Hunger fits right up there on the scale of physiological needs with air and thirst. In other words, your need to satisfy hunger is just as strong as your need to breathe or to drink water after you've been outside in the heat. It's impossible to repress that need for extended periods of time, but when you have a lot of weight to lose, that's exactly what you're asking your body to do.

Here's how it works. Ghrelin is a hormone that tells you when you're hungry. When its levels are high, you're hungry. Once you eat, your ghrelin levels go back down, and then rise again as the food digests. This is what the ghrelin levels look like for a non-dieting person at a healthy weight who eats three meals a day:

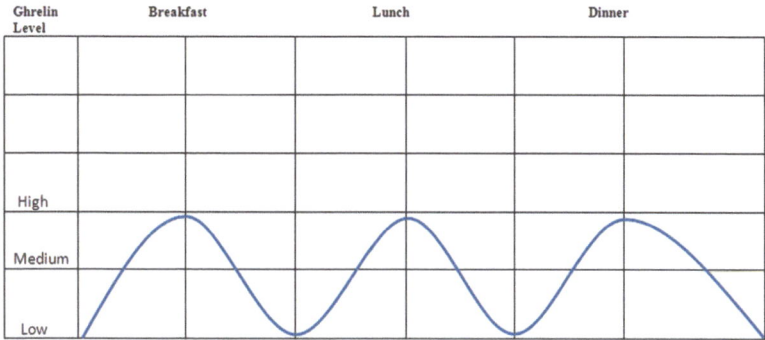

Now, let's say you need to lose a hundred pounds and you go on a sensible 1200 calorie a day diet designed to result in

a one pound per week weight loss. The red line below repre-
sents your ghrelin levels:

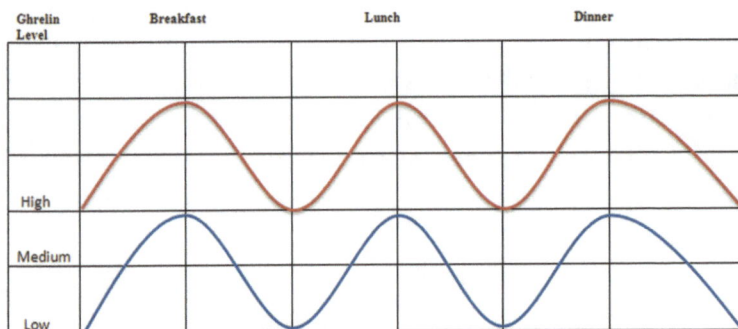

See the problem? At the fullest level, your ghrelin levels
never drop below the hunger level that would drive an average
weight person to the refrigerator. In other words, your fullest
sensation on your sensible diet is equal to the hungriest sensation of a non-dieting person at a healthy weight. No wonder so
many morbidly obese people on a diet complain that they're
always hungry. They are.

To put this in practical terms, if you want to lose one hundred pounds, you'd have to maintain a 1200 calorie a day diet
perfectly for 23 months – 734 days – a feat requiring more than
just discipline and desire. It requires hand to hand combat
with physiology that's screaming "feed me, feed me, feed me"
at you every hour of the day. It would be the same as telling
someone who's just run ten miles under a sweltering sun that
they can't have a drink of water and repeat that every day for
734 days in a row.

Even worse, you're fighting that battle with no tools other than your mind and willpower. Sure, you can go to support groups at your local Weight Watchers, but that doesn't help a whole lot at 11 o'clock at night when your stomach is growling constantly, you've been dieting for five months, and you're still 65 pounds away from a healthy weight. Suddenly the task looks impossible, and the odds that you'll leap into the car and head to the nearest fast food joint or break into your kid's stash of potato chips jump from no way to a sure thing.

That's not to say that diets never work. They can be highly effective for people who want to lose weight for the short term, like for a high school reunion or for a wedding. But no one can be on a diet for their whole lives or even for a whole year. The very terminology denotes something temporary – "I'm on a diet" indicating a limited time period, like "I'm on antibiotics". There's an expiration date.

That's not a recipe for success for permanent weight loss, because the moment you're not on the diet you gain it all back.

The only way a diet works is if it ceases to be a diet and becomes a lifestyle. But, because of the ghrelin problem, the sheer amount of weight that has to come off and the time that would require, even a lasting lifestyle change is difficult for someone with a lot of weight to lose.

In other words, option 2 – just like option 1 - also virtually guarantees an earlier death.

3. Weight loss surgery

Many look at weight loss surgery as the easy way out or some sort of too-good-to-be-true scam. In fact, it's neither.

Weight loss surgery is the only treatment for morbid obesity that offers an actual cure. Look at the percentages of weight loss outlined below for the four most common weight loss surgeries:

	Gastric Bypass	Gastric Sleeve	Lap Band	Duodenal Switch
Amount of excess weight loss[1] (number of pounds over your ideal body weight) at one year	70-77%	55%	36 to 40%	69%
Amount of excess weight loss at 2 years	77%	70%	40-50%	73-80%
Amount of weight loss maintained after 5 years	65-70% of excess weight lost	65%	60%	69-75%

Why the difference between surgery and traditional dieting? Weight loss surgery arms you with a tool for permanent weight loss that actually works.

Remember that scene in *Raiders of the Lost Ark* when the sinister looking swordsman swathed in black confronts Indiana Jones, his sword slicing through the air in a series of complicated, scary maneuvers? Just when you're sure Indiana is doomed, he pulls a gun and shoots the guy.

For most of your life, you've been fighting your morbid obesity by bringing the equivalent of a knife to a gunfight. Finally, you'll walk into the arena with a weapon that will work. Here's why.

First, all the surgeries provide portion control; i.e. you can only eat so much food at a time. Provided that you treat your altered stomach with respect, the portion control aspect of the surgery will last for the rest of your life. [3]

Second, the gastric bypass, gastric sleeve and duodenal switch surgeries bypass the part of the stomach called the gastric fundus which produces ghrelin, the hunger hormone. In other words, they take the hunger pangs off your back so that your diet can work.

The green line (gastric bypass) and orange line (gastric sleeve and duodenal switch) below represent what the ghrelin levels look like for anywhere from six to eighteen months after surgery:

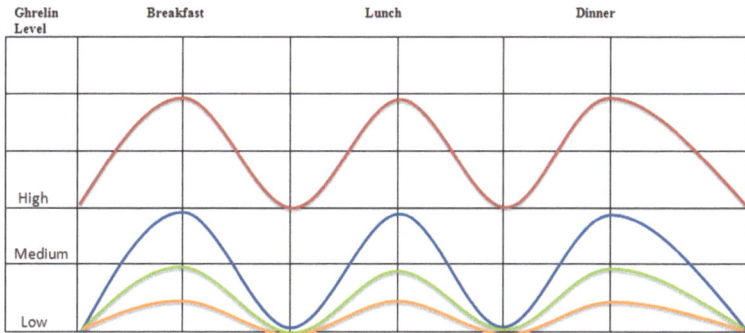

For a time, the ghrelin levels following surgery won't even reach the hunger level of a non-dieting person. This won't last forever, and other hormones will eventually come into play to

_____
3 All surgeries can be undone with concerted effort by the patient, which will be discussed in Chapter 8.

make up for the lower ghrelin levels. However, the surgeries can trick your physiology for long enough to allow you to lose a significant amount of weight, giving you time to get in the behavior modification groove of less food, more exercise, and the development of habits designed to last you the rest of your life.

Lowering ghrelin levels won't address your head hunger - emotions that make you want to eat when you're not actually hungry - but it's a useful tool. During the six to nine month period of maximum ghrelin suppression you'll learn what it feels like to "need" food versus "want" food. You'll be at the controls of your own biofeedback laboratory, getting the knack of reading the signals your body sends you when it's low on glucose and needs fuel without the noise of a faulty ghrelin message clouding the communication.

Third, the gastric bypass and duodenal switch surgeries are malabsorptive surgeries. When you eat, your food passes from your stomach through the small intestine, which is intentionally lengthy – about 22 feet. The time spent in the small intestine allows the food to be diluted and absorbed for distribution. In the gastric bypass and duodenal switch surgeries, the length of small intestine that the food passes through is reduced, meaning that less nutrients and calories are harvested from it. This is a permanent effect of the surgery.

Of the three options – doing nothing, dieting, or surgery - weight loss surgery looks like the treatment of choice.

That doesn't mean you should rush out and get it.

Let's say you have your gall bladder removed. All that's required of you is that you eat nothing after midnight, show up in the morning for the surgery, follow the post recovery instructions, and you're done. You don't ever have to think about your gall bladder again.

Weight loss surgery is just the beginning of a lifelong behavior change. You'll have to think about your weight for the rest of your life. The surgery makes the behavior change realistically possible, but you still have to put in the work.

It's the same as a professional athlete like Tiger Woods. He's phenomenally talented at golf and has been playing since he could walk. But even all his talent won't let him win without practice. He puts in 7 to 8 hours of golf practice and two to three hours of cardio, stretching and weight-lifting every day to hone his innate gift. Without the practice, even his prodigious talent wouldn't be enough to win tournaments.

Weight loss surgery provides the equivalent of the talent, but you've got to provide the work.

If you're committed to losing weight and staying healthy, your weight loss surgery will be successful. Period.

It's your only real option.

CHAPTER FOUR

Arming Yourself With The Right Weapon

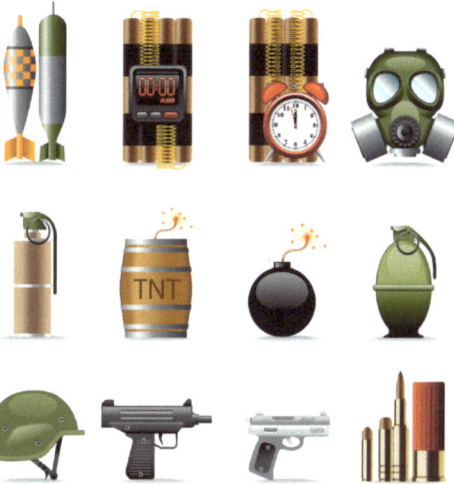

Ever try to hammer a nail into the wall using a saw? That sounds laughable, but choosing the wrong weight loss surgery for your individual characteristics will be just about as effective. There's a reason for the choices offered in weight loss surgery - what works for one person may not work for another.

Selecting the right procedure requires rigorous honesty about your lifestyle, eating habits, support system and time. Every person is different, which is why the lap band that worked for your sister might not provide the same results for you.

As you read through the details of the procedures, you'll begin to get an idea of what kind of facts you should tell your surgeon and which choice might be best for you. But no surgery, no matter how carefully chosen, will work if you're not committed to a lifelong behavior change. Getting surgery just because your spouse is nagging you to do it or your doctor prescribes it for you will end in failure. The only one who can walk this journey is you, and if you're not ready for it, no surgery will magically make up for your lack of commitment.

You'll have four surgeries to choose from – the lap band, the gastric bypass, the gastric sleeve and the duodenal switch. Each provides certain benefits, and the operation you and your surgeon select will be based on which one will give you the biggest leg up in your weight loss battle.

Here are the ways in which they can help you lose weight:

1. Portion control, meaning you can't eat as much;

2. Appetite suppression, meaning that for a period of time after the surgery you won't feel hungry because the part of your stomach that produces the hunger hormone, ghrelin, has been bypassed;

3. Malabsorption, meaning that as the food moves through your small intestines there is less time for digestion and therefore less calorie absorption; and

4. Behavior modification, meaning that if you eat too much or the wrong kinds of food, you'll feel anywhere from uncomfortable to sick, at least for some period of time after the surgery.

All the surgeries are usually done by a laparoscope under general anesthesia. In other words, instead of one long incision, between one to six small incisions are made in the abdomen, and a small lighted tube attached to a camera is guided through them. Carbon dioxide is pumped into the cavity to give a clearer visual and allow more room for the surgeon to work. The abdomen is viewed on a camera in the operating room, and long, thin instruments are used to move the organs around and perform the surgery, which means the surgeon doesn't have to cut through muscle, shortening your recovery time.

Lap Band
(Portion Control)

Lap bands came into wide use in the early 2000's and are what most people think of when they hear the words "weight loss surgery". A band lined with what acts as a high tech inflatable balloon is placed around the top of the stomach and is connected to tubing that leads to a port inserted under your skin. In most people, the port can't be seen, but if sufficient weight is lost, the port will look like a grape under the skin.

Adjustable Gastric Band (Lap Band)

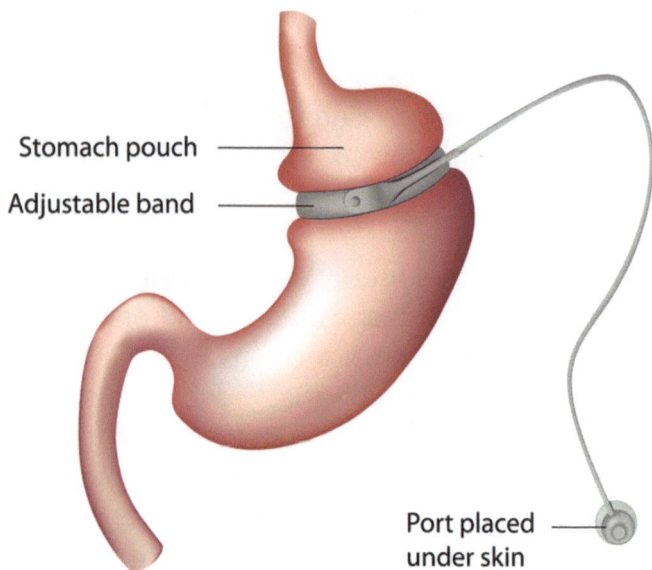

Stomach pouch

Adjustable band

Port placed
under skin

The operation takes from 20 minutes to an hour and a half, and many are performed as day surgeries. Most people are back at work at a desk within seven to ten days after surgery, and are fully recovered in four to six weeks.

How it works

Saline is injected into the port, which goes through the tubing to the balloon, inflating it around the top of your stomach like a belt. Your diminished stomach can't hold nearly as much food, and when you eat the upper part of the stomach stretches, giving a feeling of fullness.

Picture the upper part of the stomach that is now banded off as a funnel. If you put too much food too fast in the funnel, it overflows, or, in this case, makes you feel like you need to throw up.

Complications

- Lap band surgery has about the same risks as having your gall bladder removed and is lower risk than a C section. It has a one to two percent chance of: (a) infection of the band, (b) the band making a hole into the stomach, and (c) the band slipping and causing obstruction of the stomach or small bowel.

Who it works for

- People whose main issue with food is portion control.

- Those who will come in twice a month for the first 12 to 18 months to have the band adjusted.

- People who are okay with a slower weight loss.

Who it won't work for

- People whose nemesis is high calorie liquids or sugars. If you love ice cream and milkshakes, or your problem isn't so much portion control as it is the high calorie type of food you eat (like candy or desserts) this isn't the procedure for you. You'll be able to cheat from the second you leave your surgeon's office.

- People who can't commit to see their doctor twice a month for the first 12 to 18 months to have the band adjusted. This means that if you travel a lot, you can't get the time off from work to come in, or you're the type of person who has trouble keeping appointments, this is not the surgery for you.

- People who choose it because they believe it's the least invasive of the choices or that it's reversible. If you start out thinking this way, odds are you're already looking for a way out, and although the band is removable, your stomach will have scar tissue and possible effusions; i.e. liquid build-up in the abdomen. In other words, removal of the band won't leave your stomach the same as it was before the surgery.

- People who have significant health issues caused by their obesity and/or have a lot of weight to lose, since the rate of weight loss is slower than the other procedures.

Gastric Sleeve
(Portion Control and Appetite Suppression)

The gastric sleeve surgery got its origins in anti-reflux surgery, in which muscles of the esophagus were surgically corrected to stop gastric reflux. The surgery has evolved over the past twenty years into a weight loss surgery that's rapidly gaining in popularity.

The surgery consists of five laparoscopic incisions and takes thirty minutes to an hour. The stomach is resected, or cut, and then sewn or stapled into the shape of a sleeve on a garment.

Vertical Sleeve Gastrectomy

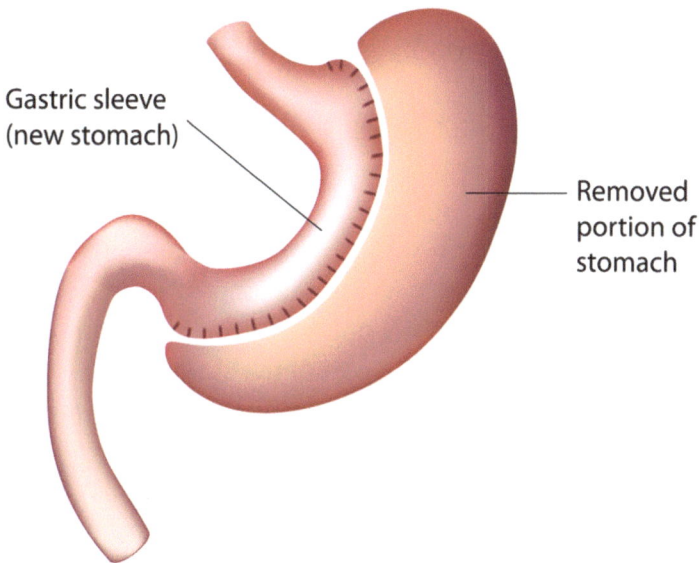

Gastric sleeve
(new stomach)

Removed
portion of
stomach

Some are done as day surgeries, while others may require a one to two night hospital stay. You'll be back at a desk job in seven to ten days, and back to normal in six weeks.

How it works

The stomach has been taken from a 64 ounce capacity down to a four to six ounce narrow tube, which means that you can't eat nearly as much. You won't get sick if you do, but you'll feel very uncomfortable. The surgery also does away with the part of your stomach that produces the hunger hormone, ghrelin, so you won't feel hungry for the first six to eighteen months.

Complications

- The operation is safer than a routine Caesarean operation, and is the safest of all the weight loss surgeries.

- It has a 1 in a 1000 chance of a leak in the staple line of the newly shaped stomach which goes away once the staple line has healed.

- Some people will have to take multi-vitamins for the rest of their lives because, depending on the person, the surgery may remove the part of the stomach that's responsible for absorbing nutrients necessary for red blood cells. Women of child bearing age while having periods will need to take multi-vitamins and vitamin B-12, and there's a 50% chance that you'll need to take a multi-vitamin supplement regardless of your age or sex.

- Some patients will experience hair loss, which is caused by rapid weight loss. It's usually only noticeable to the patient, and stops a year to a year and a half after the surgery.

Who it works for

- People whose major problem is portion control, not sweets and fatty foods.

- People who have a very high BMI which makes them risky candidates for any surgery or anyone with significant health issues that dictate a lower risk surgery.

- People who have intestinal or bowel disease and therefore are not candidates for any surgery that bypasses part of the small intestine.

Who it won't work for

- If you're a "grazer" and spend your day snacking, a vertical sleeve won't prevent that.

- If you're a sweet-a-holic, this surgery won't have any effect on your sugar habit.

Gastric Bypass (the Roux-En-Y)
(Portion Control, Malabsorptive, Appetite Suppression, Behavior Modification)

Gastric bypass came into use over a hundred years ago as a reconstructive surgery for people who'd had a traumatic stomach injury like a gunshot wound, cancer or severe ulcers. Doctors noticed that for a few months after surgical repair of the injury, patients didn't feel hungry and lost a significant amount of weight. Ultimately, the light bulb clicked on and the procedure started being used as a weight loss surgery.

The stomach is divided into a larger and a smaller portion, and then the smaller section is sewn or stapled together to make a small pouch. The pouch is then disconnected from the first part of the small intestine and reconnected to a portion slightly further down, bypassing about seven or eight feet of the intestine.

Roux-en-Y Gastric Bypass (RNY)

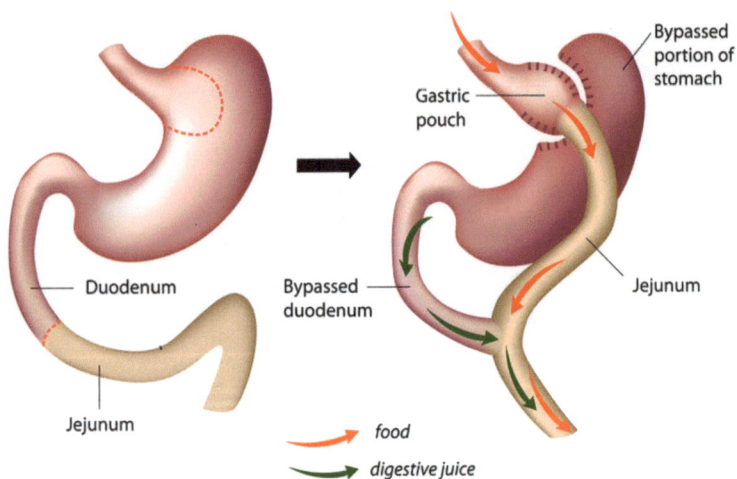

The surgery takes forty-five minutes to two hours and requires a one to two night hospital stay. You'll be back at a desk job in one and a half to two weeks, and should be fully recovered in four to six weeks.

How it works

The surgery does four things. First, the stomach size has shrunk from the size of a football, about 64 ounces, down to the size of an egg, or one to two ounces. If you eat more than the pouch can hold, you'll feel a pain or discomfort in your chest and will probably throw up.

Second, the portion of the stomach that makes ghrelin has been bypassed, so you won't feel hungry for anywhere from six to eighteen months after the surgery.

Third, your food used to go from the stomach into the upper part of the small intestine, which diluted the food with five to seven liters of bile and fluid before it traveled downstream. After surgery, the food hits the middle part of the small intestine without being diluted, meaning that if you eat processed sugars or fatty foods, your intestines will secrete hormones trying to dilute what's there. In doing so, it sucks water out of your vascular system, causing you to feel jittery and flushed, and you'll have crampy abdominal pain and explosive diarrhea and/or vomiting.

In other words, you'll feel horrible for twenty to sixty minutes. This phenomenon is called dumping syndrome and won't last for more than eighteen to twenty-four months, but while you've got it, you'll avoid any food that could trigger it.

Fourth, since part of the small intestine has been bypassed, there's less time for calorie absorption as the food travels through your intestines.

Complications

- Gastric bypass has a 1 in a 1000 chance of leaking, and a lifelong, but small, risk of an intestinal obstruction requiring a re-routing of the small intestine.

- Some patients will experience hair loss, which is a normal side effect of rapid weight loss. It's usually only noticeable to the patient, and stops a year to a year and a half after the surgery.

- Finally, you'll need to take vitamins for the rest of your life because the portion of the stomach responsible for absorbing nutrients necessary for red blood cells has been bypassed.

Who it works for

- People who have severe Type II Diabetes. Patients can see a cure or marked improvement in their diabetes in a very short period of time, normally only a few weeks.

- People whose dietary downfall is food high in sugars or fat.

- People who need portion control.

Who it won't work for:

- People who count on the behavioral modification aspects of the surgery to save them from themselves for the rest of their lives. The dumping syndrome will ultimately go away, and if you counted on it to curb your problem eating forever, you'll find yourself back in the surgeon's office having regained most or all of your weight back.

Duodenal Switch
(Portion Control, Appetite Suppression, Malabsorption, Behavior Modification)

The duodenal switch is the most severe of the weight loss surgeries, and combines aspects of both the gastric bypass and gastric sleeve surgeries. A portion of the stomach is removed and a sleeve is fashioned as in the gastric sleeve surgery, but, in addition, the majority of the small intestine is bypassed (unlike the gastric bypass which just bypasses about a third of the intestine), leaving only about three feet to be used for digestion.

Duodenal Switch

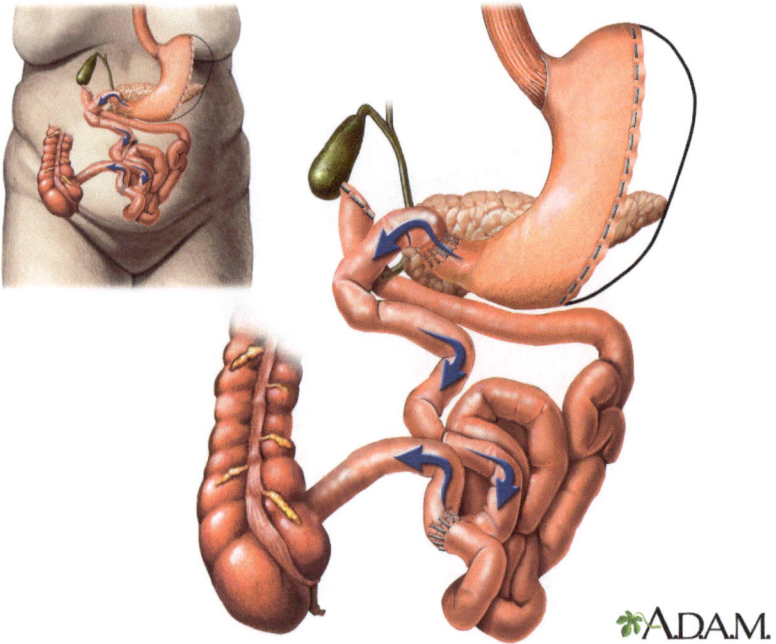

You should be back at work at a desk job in two weeks, and fully recovered in four to six weeks.

How it works

This surgery works in the same way as the gastric bypass, shrinking the size of the stomach, bypassing the ghrelin, preventing you from eating sugary or fatty foods because of the dumping syndrome and inhibiting calorie absorption because food spends less time in the small intestine. The major difference between it and the gastric bypass surgery is the dramatic effect of using only three feet of intestine to digest food.

Complications

- This surgery has a higher complication rate than any other.

- Until the stomach heals, there is a 1 in a 1000 risk of leaking, and there's a lifelong risk of intestinal obstruction.

- You'll be on vitamin and mineral supplements for the rest of your life, and failure to take them religiously can result in severe vitamin and mineral abnormalities.

- You'll have more frequent bowel movements (two to five or more per day) and very smelly gas.

- Some patients will experience hair loss, which is a normal side effect of rapid weight loss. It's usually only noticeable to the patient, and stops a year to a year and a half after the surgery.

Who it works for

- People who are severely obese, with a BMI over 50.

- People who can't stop eating and aren't going to, similar to a drug addict who has been to rehab unsuccessfully fifteen times and is going to die in the very near future.

Who is doesn't work for

- 95% of morbidly obese people. This is an extreme operation which should only be utilized by those who are severely obese and have no other good options.

The surgeries have different weight loss rates, percentages of success, and impacts on diseases caused by morbid obesity. Here's a chart summarizing the differences:

Arming Yourself With The Right Weapon

	Gastric Bypass	Gastric Sleeve	Lap Band	Duodenal Switch
Amount of excess weight loss[2] (number of pounds over your ideal body weight) at one year	70-77%	55%	36 to 40%	69%
Amount of excess weight loss at 2 years	77%	70%	40-50%	84%
Amount of weight loss maintained after 5 years	65-70% of excess weight lost	65%	60%	69-75%
Percent of patients who see cure or improvement in diabetes	96%	80-93%	77%	99%
Percent of patients who see cure or improvement in high blood pressure	90%	75%	70%	90%
Ghrelin suppression	Yes	Yes	No	Yes
Difficulty in eating processed sugar (dumping syndrome)	Yes	No	No	No
Portion control	Yes	Yes	Yes	Yes
Malabsorption (not absorbing as many calories in small intestine)	Yes	No	No	Yes
Behavior Modification	Yes	Yes	Yes	Yes

Weight Loss Surgery

Selecting the wrong surgery for your particular food issues and weight loss goals can doom you to failure. Be rigorously honest with yourself and your surgeon, and you'll pick the surgical weapon that will enable you to win your weight loss war.

CHAPTER FIVE

Hiring Your Commander-In-Chief

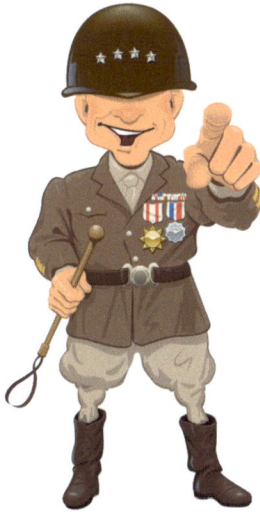

Major medical centers, ambulatory surgical centers and foreign hospitals specializing in medical tourism now offer weight loss surgery, so there's plenty to choose from. The sheer number of options can be mind-boggling. But you need to scrutinize your choices with a merciless eye. Selecting the wrong surgeon can lead to a heart breaking failure.

Medical centers may wave around the most advertising money to attract your attention, but could be staffed with general surgeons who've just recently made the switch to bariatric surgery and are far more familiar with removing gall bladders than the intricacies of and follow-up needed for successful weight loss surgery.

Foreign hospitals may offer the best price, a beautiful hotel package and throw in a spa day, but you'll be on your own once you get on the plane to head home. When you need help one, two or twenty-four months down the road, they'll be of no help unless you're able to travel and spend more money.

You need to look hard at the surgeon and his/her practice. Do your research and see at least two or three before you make your decision, because the person you choose will be in your life for years and can make or break your weight loss efforts. Picking the right one is easy if you follow these simple rules.

First, your surgeon should have done at least 1000 bariatric surgeries. If he/she hasn't, scratch that one off your list.

Second, check with the state medical board where you live to ensure that the physician is licensed. The Federation of State Medical Boards has a listing of addresses and telephone numbers for all state medical boards here: http://www.fsmb. org/directory_smb.html. For a nominal fee, the Federation will also provide you with information on whether a specific doctor's license has ever been revoked or suspended and whether he/she has ever been the subject of disciplinary action here: http://s1.fsmb.org/docinfo/. If there's no record of the doctor or they've had problems in their past, move onto the next candidate.

Third, read online reviews. Although anyone can write a review and some cranky impossible-to-please person may bash a surgeon, you shouldn't ignore numerous bad reviews, especially those that seem to have a common thread of complaint.

Fourth, interview the entire practice, not just the surgeon. Is the receptionist friendly, does the nutritionist treat you with care, is the physician's assistant competent? You'll most likely be dealing with your doctor's staff as much as the doctor, so you need to feel comfortable with them. If you're a new patient and you feel like you're in a cattle call, how do you think you'll be treated when you call at two in the morning trying to get through to your physician? If the whole practice doesn't treat you with compassion, competence and respect, then move on.

Fifth, don't rely exclusively on your general practitioner's recommendation. Most are competent to say other patients have had a good experience with a certain doctor, but they aren't competent to say how that doctor acts at the hospital. Your G.P. may not know if a particular surgeon throws things in the operating room, treats the staff with disrespect that bleeds down to the patient, or views their patients as just one more surgery in a volume practice instead of a person with a name and unique problems. The G.P.'s recommendation can be a good starting point, but shouldn't be the end of your inquiry.

Sixth, check out whether the practice meets the expectations it created. When you went for your appointment, did you see who you thought you were going to see or were you fobbed off onto someone else? Were your questions answered or were you rushed through the process? If anything feels fishy to you, walk away.

Seventh, does the practice provide access to nutritionists, psychologists and support groups to help you after the surgery? Many surgeons may not offer these services directly, but they should provide referrals to competent nutritionists and psychologists and have a close working relationship with them. If they don't, you can rest assured that the practice is focused more on their net earnings than on their patients' long term success.

Eighth, do not have surgery outside the country, no matter how great a deal they're offering. Foreign medical standards are different, you rarely get to interview the doctor before you show up for surgery, and it can be difficult to get accurate information from the governing medical body of the country as to any problems the surgeon may have had in the past. Further, if you have any complications when you get home, you'll end up in an emergency room with a doctor you don't know, who can't talk to your surgeon. Finally, you'll need ongoing support from your surgeon and his staff to be successful, which will be impossible if they're in another country.

Ninth, if and only if, more than one doctor meets the basic criteria outlined above, go with the one that makes you feel the most comfortable. Just like a woman who hates men should never go to a male gynecologist, you shouldn't choose someone who makes you feel uneasy. You won't trust what they say, which will add an extra level of difficulty to an already arduous task.

If you want someone who reminds you of your grandfatherly childhood doctor, you'll never have confidence in a younger doctor no matter how competent or highly recommended they are. If you can't trust a doctor unless he/she wears a white coat and uses big words, you won't be as likely to listen to one who uses simple words combined with a down-to-earth manner. If you believe that only Ivy League medical schools turn out competent physicians, you won't be happy with a doctor who graduated from a state medical school.

It doesn't matter whether the personal characteristics you prefer are right or wrong, logical or illogical, politically correct or not. You're about to engage in a long-term, committed relationship, and if you don't take your own personal likes and dislikes into account, the relationship will be handicapped from the start, which is no way to start a weight loss journey.

Once you've applied these nine rules, you'll find the doctor who can give you the best shot at meeting your goals and who'll still be around ten years down the road to keep congratulating you on your success.

CHAPTER SIX

Paying For Your Army

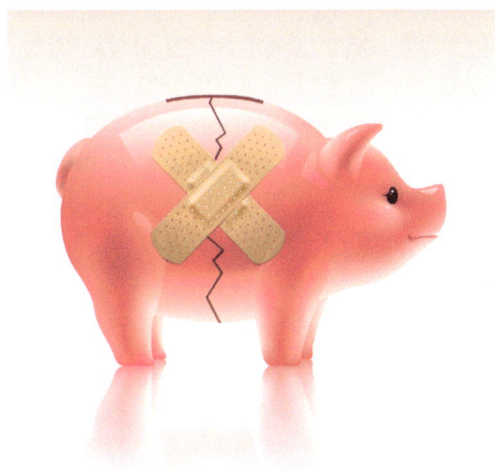

Tricky.

There's no other word for it. Whether you have health insurance or are figuring out how pay for it yourself, you'll need the wisdom of Solomon to succeed.

Bariatric surgery can wreck your family's budget even with insurance coverage. And the sheer process of qualifying for the procedure is so daunting that it's listed as one of the major reasons people don't get weight loss surgery.

So, save yourself some grief and find a surgeon who is willing to help you figure out how to pay for it without taking out a second mortgage and who will shepherd you through the process. Otherwise, you may conclude that weight loss surgery is beyond your financial and logistical reach when, in fact, a knowledgeable surgeon can help you get what you need.

The Insured Patient

Insured people thank their lucky stars they have health insurance and many times think the process will be easy, or at least as easy as insurance ever gets. Wrong. Both procedural and financial pitfalls can discourage even the most dedicated patient.

The Process

First, your insurance company may have different criteria for determining whether you're a candidate for weight loss surgery than your doctor does. For example, most insurance companies require a BMI of at least 40, or a BMI of at least 35 if you have one or more obesity-related health issues like diabetes or high blood pressure.

So what happens if you have diabetes but your BMI is only 34? Your surgeon would tell you that you're a definite candidate, but your insurance company may not agree. In that case, you may have to resort to footing the cost of the surgery yourself.

Second, your insurance company will require certain things before they'll do anything other than open a file with your name on it. Some insurers require you to go on a doctor-supervised diet for three months regardless of how many diets you've been on in the past.

Others will require a five year documented history of morbid obesity. This requirement isn't bad in and of itself, but let's say you've been obese for most of your life but only crossed into the world of morbid obesity two years ago. You'll have to wait three more years for the weight loss surgery while the damage to your body continues. You may acquire diabetes or high blood pressure during that three years which may provide the necessary health condition to qualify you for immediate surgery, but you may not want to put off surgery until the damage to your body becomes significant enough to manifest itself in a life-threatening disease. And who would blame you for that?

Third, all insurance companies require a psychological evaluation. Don't worry - it's not anyone's intent to keep you from having the surgery. Rather, the purpose is to determine whether there's a legitimate reason that surgery might actually be harmful for you.

Things that will cause a psychologist to pay close attention are eating disorders such as bulimia or night eating syndrome (in which you clean out the refrigerator at night without knowing it); mental illness that isn't properly addressed by medication, such as an untreated bipolar disorder; or something like major depression in which eating is your only coping mechanism and is the one thing that's keeping you from harming yourself.

Meeting all your insurance company's requirements can take anywhere from two to nine months, and you're going to want help. That's where a surgeon with a knowledgeable, helpful office staff can be invaluable.

Is your surgeon's office willing to file your insurance and work with the company to help you obtain coverage? Are you going to have to track down the dietician or psychologist yourself or will the surgeon's office provide you with one and help schedule the appointment? If your job hours aren't flexible, will the surgeon, dietician or psychologist see you over your lunch hour or on evenings or weekends?

Plenty of experienced surgeons provide these services. Find one who does instead of attempting to fly solo in the qualification round or you may drop out of the process before you even get started.

Sticker Shock - How Much You're Going to Have to Pay

Let's say you've jumped through all the hoops and your insurance company has authorized the procedure.

Don't relax yet.

How much you'll have to pay out of pocket depends on your deductible, whether the hospital your surgeon selects is in or out of your insurance network, and your co-pay, all of which can and should be negotiated if you find yourself raiding your kids' college fund for surgery money.

Check on your deductible – how much is it and is there one that's specific to bariatric surgery? You may think you know what your deductible is, then be stunned to learn that a totally different, and higher, one applies to weight loss surgery.

If the deductible is substantial, find out whether your surgeon and/or hospital makes you pay it up front and, if so, whether they'll accept a percentage of the deductible instead of the whole thing.

Next, ask if the hospital used by the surgeon is in-network or out-of-network, and if it's out-of-network how much extra is that going to cost you? Does the surgeon have hospital privileges at an in network hospital and will he/she schedule you in that hospital at your request?

For patients who must pay a percentage of the fees, such as on an 80/20 policy, find out when you'll have to pay the 20%. Some patients show up at the hospital the morning of their surgery and find out for the first time that they're required to write a check for their deductible and their twenty percent on the spot.

Your doctor may have some control over the hospital he or she uses, and may use more than one hospital or surgical center. Many doctors are able to negotiate better deals for their patients with the hospitals they use, particularly those with an established or higher volume practice. If you find yourself getting the bad news that you're going to owe a substantial amount of out of pocket expenses, ask whether there's a less expensive hospital you can use.

Finally, does your surgeon or the hospital provide financing for the deductible and co-pay charges or will they help you obtain financing through a third party? Many surgeons and hospitals provide very affordable financing. If yours doesn't, look around for one who does.

There's usually a way to lower the cost and obtain financing for the amount you need. Don't let the first number you hear scare you away from pursuing the procedure, and lean on your surgeon to help you find an affordable alternative.

You've Got Insurance But Bariatric Surgery is Excluded

Some policies have specific bariatric surgery exclusions, but this doesn't necessarily mean you can't get insurance coverage for the surgery.

Find a bariatric surgeon who offers insurance specialists and let them deal with the insurance company. You may mistakenly believe, based on own your reading of the policy that bariatric surgery is out of the question, but be pleasantly surprised to learn that your surgeon's insurance professionals have been able to find coverage for you.

Further, if you have a self-funded plan through your company, it's possible that you can gain approval for the surgery. In theory, the administrator of a self-funded plan can approve any surgery. A surgeon who's willing to go to bat for you with the administrator could make the case that surgery will save the plan money in the long run, and obtain the necessary green light for the procedure.

You Don't Have Insurance

Let's say you're afraid to even think about weight loss surgery because you don't have insurance and you're sure you can't afford it. Don't quit just yet.

Before you take weight loss surgery totally off the table, ask friends and other people around town how they managed to get the surgery. If you notice that three or four of your co-workers have had surgery, ask how they did it. Your company may have made arrangements, such as allowing them to borrow against a 401K.

If that's not an option, explore how much the surgery will cost if you pay cash. Many weight loss surgeons provide a discount for cash, and that price usually won't be on their website. Call and ask, and be sure and find out in detail what that price covers.

Check on whether the quoted cost covers anesthesia, pre-operative testing, sending any specimens to pathology, and follow-up appointments. If it doesn't, find out how much those services cost. Your surgeon or his/her staff should be able to tell you every service that's required, whether it's included, and if not, how much it will cost over their cash price.

Once you have a price, ask who is doing your surgery. Some practices charge more for a senior surgeon than for a junior one. The younger surgeon is probably just fine, but you don't want to be surprised on surgery day and you should research him/her as discussed in Chapter Five.

Then find out where the surgery will take place. Brand name hospitals typically charge more than lesser known ones or surgical centers. Your doctor may do his cash pay surgeries at the less expensive hospital where he/she has negotiated a better price. The cheaper hospital may be just as good as the more expensive one, but it's something you need to know when evaluating your options.

What if you don't have the cash to fully pay for the surgery, even with the discount? Ask if your surgeon offers financing. Many surgeons do, and you should be able to find one.

Finally, you don't have to stay local if the alternative is not too far away and the price is better. Surgeons in a large metropolitan area may be able to offer better prices and financing than those in smaller cities. If you live within a drivable distance, check those out. Some surgeons even offer free overnight stays in local hotels for patients traveling over a certain distance, and even that can be modified in your favor.

For those who need the surgery, there's almost always a way to make it happen with a knowledgeable, helpful surgeon.

CHAPTER SEVEN

When To Declare War

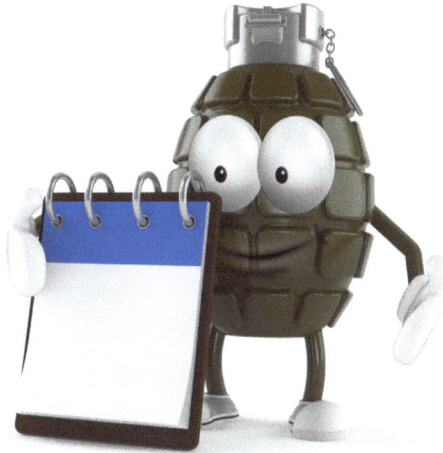

You've figured out the best way to pay for your surgery and received all the approvals required. Let's do this thing!

Hold your horses. First you need to figure out the best time to have the surgery, looking at pre- and post-surgery issues, as well as what's happening emotionally in your life and the impact your surgery will have on others around you.

Most patients don't just show up on the day of surgery having had to do nothing other than pack their jammies. They've been on a two to three week special diet designed to shrink their liver so their surgeon can operate on them safely.

So what's on your schedule for the weeks right before surgery?

If you're going on a Caribbean cruise, a Napa Valley wine tour, or attending your daughter's rehearsal dinner and wedding, then this is not the time to be on a pre-op diet. No matter what you tell yourself, you won't be able to stick to the doctor approved menu plan.

And if your liver is too big, the surgeon may stop in the middle of surgery and close you back up. Then, you'll have to start over again, and if you're using insurance, you may run into problems with obtaining approval for scheduling a second surgery when you didn't modify your behavior for the first.

As to your post-op plans, you'll need to leave yourself enough time from both work and family commitments to recover.

The amount of time your doctor tells you that you need to take off from work will depend on your job. If you work from home on a computer, you could be back at it in two to three days. If you have a desk job, you should plan to return to work in ten to fourteen days. If you're a fireman, you may not be back at work for four to six weeks.

Take your doctor's word on this. It doesn't matter how tough you are or that you've always been a fast healer. The recovery time is based on your surgeon's experience with thousands of people, some just as strong and quick to recover as you are. The worst thing you can do is over-promise and under-deliver to your boss, your clients, your kids, your spouse or your co-workers.

Once you know when you can realistically be back at work, think about whether you can take that time off. You don't want to emerge from weight loss surgery healthier but jobless. If you don't have the medical leave or vacation time built up that you need, it might be worth waiting six months until you do.

If you're a stay-at-home mom, how old are your kids, how active are they, and how much help will you need in taking care of them? If they can't take care of themselves, who will help you, and are the helpers available for the period of time that you'll need them?

Next you need to think about whether you're emotionally ready. The initial adjustment will be stressful and your focus needs to be on yourself.

Are you going through a divorce, or adjusting to bipolar medication, or trying to finish your graduate thesis? Are you trying to boost your sales numbers for a promotion or dealing with a sick child or an ailing parent that requires your full attention?

If you are, then this is probably not the right time for weight loss surgery. The surgery and the accompanying behavioral changes will be hard enough, and upping the degree of difficulty can ruin your chances for success. The wiser course might be to wait until things calm down a bit.

The final bit of preparation that's totally up to you is figuring out whether you want anyone to know about your surgery. Some people are perfectly comfortable with opening up about their surgery, while others would die before they'd tell. If you fall in the latter category, you need to give careful thought to the reason you're going to use for your absence from work or social commitments.

If you tell someone you're having your gall bladder out and then have gall stones three months later, you'll be officially busted. Pick something boring like reflux surgery or exploratory laparoscopic surgery to evaluate abdominal pain. Those are far less likely to trip you up.

If the person taking care of you is your mother but you don't want her to know you're having weight loss surgery, you need to re-think that decision or find another caregiver. Your odds of fooling her rank somewhere below sighting the Loch Ness monster in your backyard pool.

If you're going to be in the hospital overnight and are expecting guests, you need to make sure that hospital staff knows not to ask about your gastric bypass in front of your co-workers. If you're keeping the nature of the surgery a secret, the better option is to tell those who need to know that you're having day surgery and your doctor says you won't be up to visitors for three or four days.

Once you've planned what to tell others and have figured out that your work, family and emotional situation will allow for the surgery, then you'll be in the final phase.

You'll probably have a pre-surgery appointment with your doctor, who will check to see if your medications or health condition has changed. Typically, you'll have some routine blood work done, and then, depending on your risk factors, you may have an EKG, an evaluation of your stomach or intestines in the form of x-rays (an upper GI) and an endoscopy. Some people may need to get clearance from a heart and lung doctor. If you haven't already, you'll go to the dietitian to discuss whether you need to be on a special diet before surgery.

Your doctor and possibly your hospital will load you down with information packets. Look them over carefully to make sure they don't contradict each other. If they do, ask your surgeon which one you should follow.

The surgery itself is in your doctor's hands. But once you go home, your success rests in your hands. Take a deep breath – now the real journey begins.

CHAPTER EIGHT

Don't Handcuff Your Army

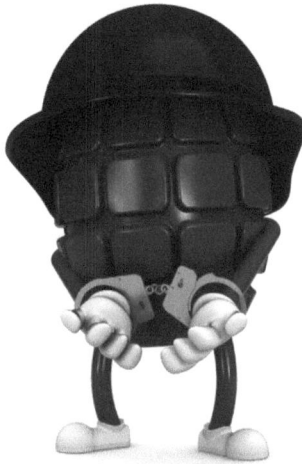

In 1876, the Gatling Gun changed the face of warfare. It could fire 300 rounds per minute and was the precursor to the modern machine gun. When General Custer set off toward Little Big Horn, he left the Gatling Guns behind, partly because he just didn't think it would be sporting to use such a guaranteed battle winner against the poor Sioux Indians.

At some point during the massacre of his men, Custer must have thought, "If only I'd brought the Gatling Guns…"

Your weight loss surgery will give you vital weapons to use in curing your morbid obesity. If you use them properly, you'll be cured. If you don't, you won't.

There aren't that many rules for using the weapons your surgery has given you and they aren't complicated. Following them should become second nature to you.

The Preliminary Rules – The First Four to Six Weeks

You only have three main rules to follow for the first four to six weeks after your surgery:

1. Do whatever your surgeon tells you to do.

2. Don't do whatever your surgeon tells you not to do.

3. Put only liquids in your stomach.

Rule number 3 is really just a subset of Rule Numbers 1 and 2, but failing to follow it has landed so many patients in the emergency room that it has earned special mention.

You'll be given explicit instructions in writing from your surgeon and possibly your hospital. Follow them to the letter. Your surgery is made to last you a lifetime, so give it a chance to work by doing exactly what your surgeon tells you to do.

This is not the time to substitute your mom's judgment or the advice of your best-friend-who-had-the-surgery-three-years-ago for the directions given to you by your medical professionals. And if there's any difference between what the surgeon tells you and what your hospital tells you, call your surgeon and let he/she resolve the conflict. Don't try to reconcile it yourself.

So why are you stuck with "eating" only liquids? Most patients have already been on a restrictive pre-surgery diet to shrink their liver, and hearing that they're relegated to weeks of drinking only liquids can sound like cruel and unusual punishment.

Liquids won't stress the suture or staple line on your re-shaped stomach while it's healing. Liquids are anything you can pour through a strainer, which means things like yogurt, jello, smoothies, watery mashed potatoes, or any solid food you've tried to puree into a liquid shouldn't pass your lips.

Why? Thicker liquids won't conform to the shape of your new stomach. Think of the difference between putting water and yogurt into a balloon. Water will take on the shape of the balloon, whereas the yogurt will stick to one spot and deform its shape.

The same thing will happen in your stomach if you put something in there other than a liquid that will pass through a sieve – it will glob up and could put pressure on the suture/staple line, which might cause anything from a small leak to a total rupture.

You don't want that to happen.

Keeping this rule will be pretty easy for the first two weeks. Initially, you'll feel full with only a medicine cup of liquid. The second week you won't be hungry at all.

But watch out for the third week. You'll be feeling good, you might be getting a little bored, your stomach will feel fine, and you'll conclude it must be healed.

Wrong. It takes 21 to 28 days for a suture/staple line to fully heal, no matter how fast a healer you are.

Stick to the liquids.

The good news is that once you've healed, the odds of rupture at the site of the operation are virtually none. Scar tissue forms around the suture/staple line, and it's stronger than stomach tissue.

The "'Til Death Do You Part" Rules

After you've made it to solid food, you'll have a new set of rules designed to keep the benefits of the surgery intact for the rest of your life. You won't be able to cure your morbid obesity unless you keep the "'Til Death Do You Part" Rules:

1. If it bubbles, don't put it in your mouth.

2. You're not a cow, so don't eat like one.

3. If it grows when you water it, avoid it.

4. If it ends in –ose or –ccino, just say no.

5. Don't drink so much that you can't be the designated driver.

6. Find a new best friend.

7. Recognize the beauty of "no".

8. Keep your head out of the sand.

9. Be selfish.

Rule Number 1: If it Bubbles, Don't Put It In Your Mouth.

Your surgically altered stomach will stay small if you treat it well. If you don't, it will stretch to a larger size and you'll lose the portion control feature of your operation.

Before surgery, your stomach was elastic, similar to a balloon. When you ate or drank too much, it would stretch to accommodate the load and then shrink back to its normal size as the food left the stomach.

It doesn't work that way for stomachs altered by weight loss surgery. The stomach loses its elasticity, so it won't spring back to its smaller size. If you stretch it out, it will stay stretched. It's like a sock with worn out elastic that keeps falling down around your ankles.

This means you shouldn't drink any carbonated beverage, whether that's a Coke, a club soda, champagne, bubbly water, an alcoholic drink using a carbonated base as a mixer like a mimosa or a jack and Coke, or any effervescent liquid like an Alka-Seltzer tablet mixed in water.

Here's why. When you drink a carbonated beverage, you're quadrupling the volume that has to be handled by your stomach. So if you drink a twelve ounce diet Coke, you're injecting about 48 ounces of liquid and air into a sac designed to hold 4 to 6 ounces. When a person does that who's never had bariatric surgery, they'll initially feel bloated but within minutes they'll burp and their stomach will snap back to normal.

Your stomach won't. Repeated exposure of your stomach to any carbonated liquid will ultimately ruin any weight loss surgery that provides portion control. And if you stretch your stomach, options for getting back that portion control range from limited to non-existent, depending on the procedure. In other words, the surgery will give you the best portion control you'll ever have, even if you go back and have revision surgery.

A corollary to this rule is to avoid drinking from a straw. Although not as harmful as drinking a carbonated beverage, a straw acts as a miniature carbonation machine, injecting air into what you're sipping.

Rule Number 2: You're Not a Cow, so Don't Eat Like One.

Don't graze. You can defeat your weight loss surgery by snacking all day long. It's like plugging a sink and letting a faucet drip in it for hours. The sink won't overflow because the volume of water going into the sink per minute is so little that it can accommodate it.

In the same way, you can drip food constantly into your stomach in small amounts throughout the day, dodging the portion control aspect of your surgery but dooming yourself with the calorie intake.

Be rigorous in examining what you eat. The four M&M's that you grab from the jar on your counter every time you walk by, the free cheese sample at the store, the taste of the baked goodies that your buddy brought to the office, the "just a bite" of your husband's piece of pie – you may not even count them in your calorie intake, but they all add up in your expensive, hard-earned smaller stomach.

Don't drip-drip your way into sabotaging your portion control tool.

Rule Number 3: If it Grows When You Water it, Avoid It.

Rice, pasta and bread expand when they're moistened, doubling or even tripling in size. They swell in your stomach and farther downstream at the entrance to your intestine, plugging things up for a bit and causing your stomach to enlarge while it holds up digestion of everything else until the now super-sized food can make it through. Over time, this will stretch your stomach.

Don't panic - this doesn't mean you can never eat bread or pasta or rice. It means that you should only eat it on occasion, and when you do you should eat very limited amounts.

Rule Number 4: If It Ends In –Ose or –Cino, Just Say No.

Drinks like milkshakes, fruit juices and super-sugary smoothies contain lots of glucose or fructose; i.e. sugar. Many weight loss patients looking for ways to get enough protein become mesmerized by the protein count in a drink and somehow miss the calorie count. You'll drink jacked-up protein smoothies thinking you're being healthy and wonder why your weight keeps creeping up instead of going down. Too late, you'll figure out that your favorite smoothie has as many calories as two and a half meals.

The same applies to coffee drinks. Cappuccinos and Frappuccinos pack too many calories for too little nutritional value.

But, you say, I'm only going to have one a month. Don't kid yourself. For people who like it, sugar begets more sugar, acting like natural crack cocaine. You'll find yourself going from one milkshake a month to one every two weeks to one a week to – well, you get the picture.

Don't even get started down that road. There's a reason elderly, stick-thin people are given drinks like Ensure - high calorie beverages work for people who need to gain weight. You're not one of those people.

Rule Number 5: Don't Drink So Much That You Can't Be the Designated Driver.

Immediately after surgery while you're healing, you shouldn't have any alcohol because it can cause ulcers and impede healing. But after you've finished healing, you may be able to drink alcohol on a limited basis, depending on the type of procedure you had and your body's tolerance.

A good rule of thumb? Don't drink any amount that would disqualify you from being a designated driver. That means you shouldn't have more than one drink.

For every procedure but the lap band, alcohol will affect you more after your surgery than it did before because it will be absorbed more quickly. The drink that wouldn't have had any discernable effect before surgery may knock you on your rear afterward. Over time, you may be able to drink more without as big of a reaction, and some will go back to their pre-surgery tolerance.

But ingesting more than one drink stacks up calories you don't need and starts falling into the verboten high calorie beverage category. So, if you drink at all in the years following your surgery, keep it down to one.

Rule Number 6: Find a New Best Friend.

Let's face it - food acts as an undemanding best friend that's always there, day or night, to soothe or provide blessed oblivion. Most patients don't realize the intense, emotional relationship they have with food until they wake up from surgery and can't lean on it anymore. Suddenly their best friend is gone and they don't have anything to take its place.

Exacerbating the problem is the fact that food may have also taken up a lot of your time in your pre-surgery days. After surgery, the time will still be there, and the need for comfort will still arise.

It's vital to figure out something enjoyable to fill the void and to provide the escape that food used to give you. This could be gardening, reading, prayer, meditation, walking, or a new hobby like quilting or woodcraft or flying radio-controlled airplanes.

Everyone has something they like to do, and if you don't already have a substitute to fill the hole that changing your relationship with food will leave, experiment until you find something you like.

Rule Number 7: Recognize the Beauty of "No".

Successful people say no – no to the piece of wedding cake, the champagne cocktail or the lavish helping every mother wants to put on their child's plate at Thanksgiving.

There's nothing wrong with saying "no", and it's a habit that can help you in all areas of your life. Usually, your concern about uttering the word is greater than the rejection the other person feels. If you don't take that glass of champagne at your daughter's wedding, no one is going to be upset. And on the occasions that someone does react negatively, you can explain the reason for your refusal if they are someone important to you, or laugh it off if they're not.

Saying "no" is an act of love to yourself - protecting yourself from demands others make that can hurt you. Embracing "no" in a post-surgery life is another way of embracing yourself.

Rule Number 8: Keep Your Head Out of the Sand.

Achieving and maintaining a goal requires focus. It's easy to get busy with other things after the first flush of weight loss and lose focus on maintaining a healthy weight. That's when you wake up forty, fifty or a hundred pounds later and realize you've had your head firmly in the sand while your weight crept up on you.

You can keep this from happening by finding something that keeps your weight goals at the forefront of your mind. Check out support groups, chat forums, exercise groups, daily meditation with a habitual focus for at least part of the time on maintaining a healthy weight, a daily log of how you met your goal of staying healthy on that day – anything that requires you to think about your weight goals.

That's one of the main functions of Alcoholics Anonymous meetings, particularly for those who've been sober for years.

Attending regular meetings reminds them of their journey to sobriety and the vigilance required to stay there.

It's hard to delude yourself when you have a regular activity that focuses you on your issue. Keeping your healthy weight at the forefront of your mind will help you be successful in your weight loss journey.

Rule Number 9: Be Selfish.

Remember the flight attendant's announcement before every takeoff warning parents to put the oxygen mask on themselves first before putting one on their child in the event of an emergency? At first blush, that sounds awfully selfish – what kind of a parent would do that?

But if you don't make sure you're around to care for your child during the emergency, then both of you will die. The same logic applies to staying healthy.

You may have children at home, a spouse, a demanding boss, three dogs, two horses, a gerbil and aging parents– all of whom need your help. You may feel like you're not being a good mother/wife/employee/daughter/church member if you're not giving a hundred percent to others, even if it means neglecting yourself.

But if you don't take care of yourself, you're ultimately not going to be able to take care of anyone else. You've got to put the oxygen mask on yourself first.

This requirement boils down to taking time, even if it means depriving others. You'll need time daily to exercise, time to grocery shop and cook instead of going through the fast food line, time to go to support groups or meditate or whatever you choose to do to keep your health in the forefront of your mind.

People who depend on you may initially protest. Loudly. Although most people buy into the idea of taking personal time for yourself, they usually don't think it's such a good idea when it interferes with their customary lifestyle.

Don't give in. No one will carve time out from your schedule for you – you're the only one who can do it. And it's not as though you'll take leave of all your responsibilities. The amount of time we're talking about isn't going to hurt anyone, although it may require some who haven't been carrying their load to start taking on a fair share during your momentary absences.

If this concept is difficult for you, then just tell yourself you need to break the top five. In other words, maybe you put your youngest daughter and your husband as numbers one and two, leaving yourself to come in third. That's okay. If, however, you assess what you're spending your time and energy on and find yourself coming in at sixth place or higher, you need to re-prioritize if you want to stay healthy.

Don't handcuff your army – use every tool you've got and keep them in good working order.

CHAPTER NINE

When to Call In Reinforcements

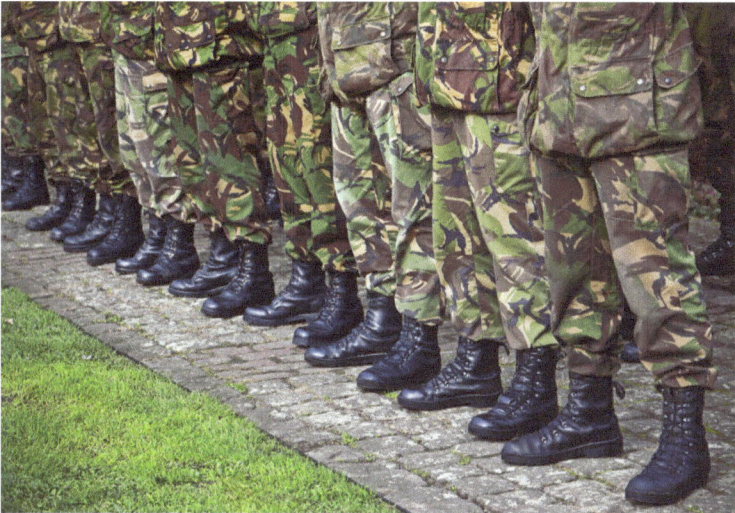

Weight loss surgery causes fewer complications than gall bladder surgery or a Caesarean section. But, they can occur, so if you're feeling sick, you need to let your doctor know. That doesn't make you a complainer or a high maintenance patient – it just makes you a smart cookie.

The three major tells that you're having a problem are nausea, vomiting and a fever of over 101 degrees Fahrenheit. Each one could be signs of a rupture, an infection, a blood clot, an internal hernia or gallstones. If you have any of those symptoms, call your surgeon, not your primary doctor or your ob/gyn or the local doc-in-the-box. And, if you possibly can, call your surgeon rather than showing up at the hospital and submitting to the judgment of whatever young doctor is manning the emergency room that night.

Many doctors aren't familiar with the most common complications of weight loss surgery, and could take hours, days, weeks or even months to figure out a problem that your weight loss surgeon would have nailed within minutes.

For example, one to two percent of patients who've had gastric bypass surgery develop an internal hernia, something which is not detectable from a CT scan. Some patients try in vain to get a diagnosis for months before they see their weight loss surgeon, who most likely could have identified the problem immediately, saving them money, time, pain and energy.

A small number of patients may develop a bowel obstruction caused by the scar tissue left from the surgery. Your surgeon can recognize the problem right away and correct it in a twenty minute procedure that will have you back to work the next day. If you see a doctor who doesn't have extensive experience with weight loss surgery, he/she may not figure out the problem in time to keep the bowel obstruction from becoming acute, at which point you're in for a more extensive surgical repair and a lengthier recovery time.

At the other end of the spectrum, many doctors will blame any abdominal pain on your weight loss surgery once they find out you've had it. Abdominal pain is not normal at any time after bariatric surgery. Your surgeon can determine quickly whether your current problem has any relationship to your surgery, and if not, can direct you to another doctor to look for the right culprit before precious time slips away.

You should feel free to call your weight loss surgeon for the rest of your life if you experience symptoms you suspect may be related to the surgery. Good surgeons won't treat your call as a bother or a nuisance, but will respond professionally and make sure you get the help you need.

CHAPTER TEN

Never Stop Drilling

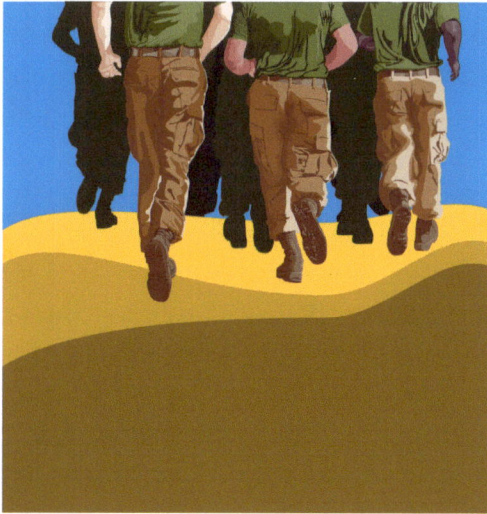

What's up with the religion of exercise? You've been told a million times that you have to exercise, but, seriously, what person in their right mind wants to do that?

Weight Loss Surgery

You've watched the faces of the contestants on The Biggest Loser go from pink to red to heart-attack-purple trying to keep up with their trainers' workout demands, and there's always one poor shlub who collapses before the session is over. On the few times you've ventured to your gym, you've seen weirdly bulging men making ugly guttural sounds as they heave free weights up to their chest. You've done your best to avoid looking at the wet spots left on the gym equipment and you breathed through your mouth so you wouldn't smell the sweat stink permeating the mats around the elliptical trainer.

Physical agony, sweat, disgusting odors, exhaustion – nothing about exercise looks appealing.

Exercise doesn't have to be like that. You can get in enough physical exertion to stay healthy and maintain your weight loss without physical pain, sweating through your clothes or going to a gym.

It's all about the 10,000 steps. Get in 10,000 steps every day, any way you can, and that's enough to boost and maintain your weight loss and improve your cardiovascular health.

Putting in 10,000 steps doesn't mean going to a gym and getting on a treadmill. If you're an exercise-a-phobe, you can get in the necessary steps by parking farther from your office building or grocery store, taking the stairs instead of the elevator up and down from floor to floor, hot-footing it to the corner store instead of driving, walking your dog, pacing the sidelines at your kids' games or taking the file to your co-worker's office instead of having someone else do it.

You'll be amazed at how the steps add up, and you'll find yourself enjoying figuring out new ways to get in your steps while doing your ordinary chores.

This means you'll need to invest in a pedometer, and it'd be a good idea to keep a daily log of how many steps you've taken each day. Keeping the log will ensure that you're keeping your health at the forefront of your mind and are thinking about ways to get in your 10,000 steps every day.

In the beginning, you may not be able to get in 10,000 steps. Don't worry – that's normal. As your weight drops and your fitness increases, you'll work up to it. Figure out your average number of steps per day and try to increase that number each week by 20% until you reach your goal.

And you don't have to be smelly, sweaty, go to a gym, or buy special clothes to do it.

Some patients will find that, despite all odds, they love exercise. They may like the way it makes them feel or the way it makes them look. They'll sign up for a 10K race, they'll discover that the runner's high really does exist, they'll like the camaraderie of the cycling group they joined or they'll make friends at the early morning boot camp workout.

It doesn't matter if you love or hate exercise, if you run a marathon or walk extra distances in your parking lot. You can exercise enough to be healthy, whether you choose to do it by incremental steps all day long or in a high-tech cycling outfit on a twenty mile ride.

And you have to do it.

It's almost impossible to maintain weight loss without exercise. Most people gain weight by eating only ten to a hundred extra calories a day, which adds up to putting on an extra one to ten pounds per year. Getting in the minimum 10,000 daily steps keeps that from happening.

If you have to call it something other than exercise to make it palatable, do it. If you need a special outfit to motivate yourself to exercise, do it. If you need to hire a trainer to walk with you, do it. If you can't stand to walk but love to shop, get your steps in by walking around the mall and window shopping.

It doesn't matter how you get it done – just do it.

CHAPTER ELEVEN

Don't Tolerate Double Agents

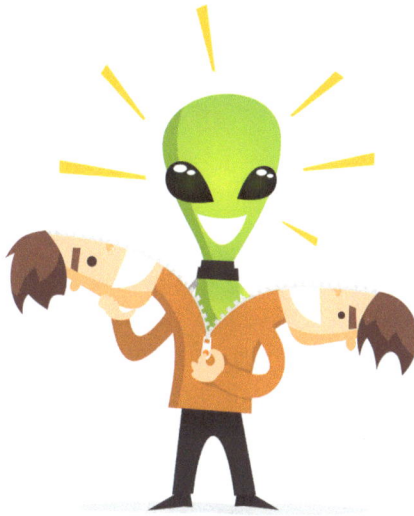

Every war has its Benedict Arnold, and yours is no different.
He'll be easy ferret out. All you've got to do is look in the mirror.
Morbid obesity is rarely about eating. It's about avoiding.

Many patients believe that their excess weight was the overriding problem in their lives, and once it's gone, everything will be better. No question their health will be better, but the excess weight was only a symptom of the problem – it was never THE problem. If they continue avoiding the real problem, sooner or later they'll eat their way out of whatever weight loss procedure they had.

People eat to avoid dealing with things they'd rather not face: pain, hurt or guilt; depression; conflict; job dissatisfaction; childhood molestation; boredom; an unhappy marriage; feelings of unworthiness; and loneliness. A shocking number of patients have no idea that they've been using food as a combination security blanket/soother/constant companion until they no longer have it available.

After your surgery, whatever you're avoiding will announce itself with a bang. On the bright side, you've just saved yourself thousands of dollars on a psychiatrist's couch. On the not-so-bright side, you've got to figure out your core issue and an effective way to deal with it – pronto - or you'll end up being the only truly effective enemy against your weight loss war.

Although everyone's reasons for becoming morbidly obese are invariably a combination of deeply rooted, complicated and unique experiences, getting rid of food as your go-to coping mechanism almost always involves facing the truth. And you're given a wonderful opportunity to ferret out the truth by examining the emotions that surface immediately after surgery when you can't use food to hide from it any longer.

For example, if you've got a job you hate and you've snacked your way through the day to cope with it and rewarded yourself for persevering with food once you got home, you may need to embrace the truth that you need to find a different job. If you're in an abusive relationship, you may need to accept the truth that he/she isn't going to change and you've got to leave that relationship, even if it means less financial security or sharing custody of your children.

There are a myriad of issues that can't be "fixed" simply by taking yourself out of the situation. If your parents constantly gave you a message of disapproval that now feels etched into your bones, you'll need to develop a new image of yourself, forgive your parents, and protect yourself from reacting to any continued toxic messaging from them. If you have a surly teenager who's constantly in trouble and you dread every phone call from a number you don't recognize, you're going to have to live in that truth instead of avoiding it, and find another coping mechanism to deal with your anxiety over your child.

Sometimes you don't know what your issue is, and, in fact, could swear you don't have one.

You do.

No one becomes morbidly obese without having some issue they're hiding from. We're all products of a long emotional road map made up of childhood experiences, social norms, invisible childhood cues, trauma, and the cards life has dealt along the way.

Figuring out and dealing with the reasons for your reliance on food as a coping mechanism needs to be number one on your to-do list.

Your surgeon can refer you to support groups, therapists and other helpful resources. You can read quality books on the topic or use a trusted friend or family member as a sounding board to help you. One way or another, you need to figure out what's causing your problem and change it, or find a different way to cope with it.

Your surgeon can operate on your stomach. It's up to you to operate on your head.

CHAPTER TWELVE

What To Do When The War Effort Stalls

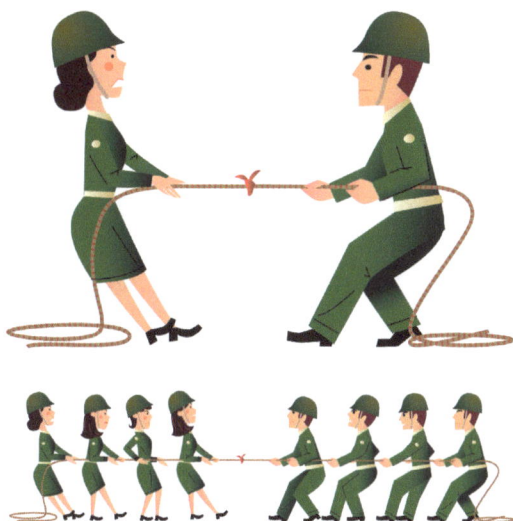

"I'm doing everything right but I've stopped losing weight."

It's a common complaint, and plateauing in your weight loss will happen.

Don't panic.

First, look at whether you really are doing everything right. You may have lost the dedicated zeal you had in your first few months or years following surgery. You focused hard on your own health after your surgery but now you've shifted your attention to other things and have become a bit less rigid about your diet and exercise.

Maybe you've been grazing during the day more than you realize, or you've added ice cream back into your repertoire now that your dumping syndrome is gone, or you're not as careful when you go out to eat as you once were. Maybe you only work out three times a week when a year ago your gym's Stairmaster practically had your name engraved on it. It won't be difficult to figure out.

Take a hard look at your habits and compare them to what you were doing before you gained the twenty or thirty pounds. If you haven't already, begin keeping a food and exercise journal and review it carefully. You'll find your weight gain culprit.

Second, you may be a victim of slowing metabolism. The average patient walks into their bariatric surgeon's office around their fortieth birthday, which means they begin their weight loss war on a battlefield of increasingly unfavorable conditions. The rate of metabolism slows in your early forties, and then falls off a cliff between ages forty-five to fifty.

If you're in that milestone decade, your body's slowing metabolic rate explains why you're eating and expending the same amount of calories you were a year ago but your weight keeps creeping up. You've got to eat less, exercise more, or do both.

Before you fall into a blue funk over the unfairness of it all, keep in mind that you've now landed in the world of mainstream weight problems. Slowing metabolism happens to everyone, even people who never had to worry about their weight before. You'll have lots of company in finding the right strategies to keep your weight down as you age.

Third, you may have succumbed to the success phenomenon. Many bariatric patients find themselves on the fast track at work, their career soaring to unexpected heights because of their weight loss and increased self-confidence. The impact of success on weight (unless you're a professional athlete) can be predicted almost to a mathematical certainty:

$$\text{Promotion} + \text{Increased Pay} + \text{More Responsibility} =$$
$$\text{Less Energy Expended} =$$
$$\text{WEIGHT GAIN}$$

Why? You get a closer parking space so you don't burn the hundred calories you once did by parking in the boonies and walking up the stairs in the parking garage. Someone now gets your files for you and people come to your office instead of you walking to theirs. You're spending longer hours sitting behind a desk or studying your computer screen. You can afford expensive wine at dinner now instead of iced tea. Someone else mows your lawn, cleans your house, walks your dog and washes your windows.

Remember the ten pounds a year just a hundred extra calories a day adds to your frame? Your very success may have resulted in small changes in your normal routine that, over time, led to the twenty or thirty pounds you've been unable to shed.

What if none of these three theories explains your weight plateau? You're eating the same amount of calories and exercising the same amount that you were, but your weekly weight loss has shrunk from ten pounds, to five, to one, and finally down to zero.

Here's what's happening.

During the first few weeks of weight loss, calories from food are reduced and the body gets needed energy by releasing its stores of glycogen, a type of carbohydrate found in the muscles and liver. Glycogen holds on to water, so when glycogen is burned for energy, it also releases water, resulting in substantial weight loss that's mostly water.

Your metabolism slows as you lose mass, so you burn fewer calories than you did at your heavier weight even doing the same activities. The fact that you're no longer getting the benefit of the water weight loss and that it takes fewer calories to support your lighter frame means that you're going to have to change the calories in/calories out equation if you want to keep losing; i.e. eat less, exercise more, or do both.

If you're trying and you can't seem to get past the weight-loss plateau or are even gaining weight, it's time to call in the professionals. Go see your bariatric surgeon and give a candid explanation of what's going on, not only with your weight, but with your life. Between the two of you, you'll find the answer, and can develop a plan to get you back to where you want to be.

Whatever you do, don't give up and go back to your old eating habits. You've already shown you can lose weight and keep it off. Once you figure out the reasons you've lost some ground, you can make the appropriate changes and get back to where you want to be.

CHAPTER THIRTEEN

Keeping the Peace: The DMZ and MDL

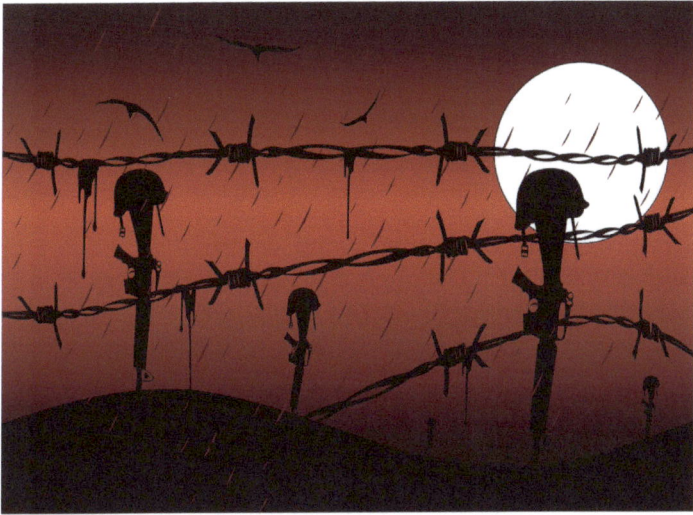

The war between North and South Korea technically ended on July 27, 1953, but every day since then both sides take up their assault rifles, keep their rocket launchers handy, and stand facing each other over a fragile buffer strip called the DMZ, or the demilitarized zone. The only military forces allowed in the DMZ are limited patrols, and they must stop on their own side of a boundary called the military demarcation line, or the MDL.

The names sound innocuous, but here's what they really mean. Venturing into the DMZ requires nerves of steel since even twitching the wrong way could cause an international incident and the real possibility of renewed war. And if you misjudge the boundary of the MDL and step an inch over the line, you'll probably be shot. Since the 1953 cease fire, over 550 people have been killed for stepping over the MCL, an average of about nine a year.

In other words, the DMZ is the danger zone and the MDL is the killing zone.

Your weight loss war is the same. You may be down to a healthy weight, but you shouldn't retire the troops. You need to create your own DMZ and MDL.

What does that mean? You should select two numbers: a weight that's your early warning signal that tells you you're in danger of giving up your hard won victory over your morbid obesity, and a weight that's your drop dead number, a number you won't cross no matter what.

You should choose those two numbers while you're still in the honeymoon stage of your weight loss, while you're still pumped up about how much better your life is and you can't even imagine going back to your old self. Write them down, and make a solemn promise to yourself that you won't ignore them. Treat that promise as seriously as you would treat a wedding vow or the unspoken promise you make to your children at their birth to take care of them.

Your DMZ weight is the one at which you'll sit down and take a hard look at your habits and get back to doing what you know to do to keep your weight in order.

Let's say you try that but you seem to keep gaining weight, or you just can't make yourself get back to a healthy lifestyle and you find yourself at your MDL. That's when you need to go see your bariatric surgeon.

It doesn't matter if you don't want to do it, or even if at that moment you don't intend to do anything about your weight. If you've got a good surgeon, he/she can talk with you about what's going on, and may be able to provide the encouragement and structure you need to get back in the groove.

A good surgeon won't be judgmental and won't berate you. Every weight loss surgeon has been in the trenches long enough to know how tough the battle can be, and they've heard your story thousands of times. They also know how to help you get back on track.

You absolutely do not want to gain your weight back because if you do, your options will be limited.

First, another weight loss surgery will hardly ever be better than the original one. If your initial surgery provided ghrelin suppression which alleviated your hunger, other hormones have up-regulated to compensate, and those can't be suppressed. If you had a procedure which resulted in dumping syndrome, your body has adapted and you can eat sweets with no adverse consequences. And although the opening to your stomach or sleeve can be tightened somewhat and the pouch reduced slightly, it will never work as well as it did in the first surgery.

Second, if you've failed at one weight loss surgery, your odds of being successful at a another one are much less for the simple reason that you know without a doubt that you can undo the surgery. While some bariatric patients are terrified they'll cause themselves physical harm if they eat too much or indulge in the wrong food, you know eating your way out of your surgery won't kill you – at least not immediately.

Third, unless you had a mechanical problem; i.e. the procedure or device itself was flawed, you didn't really buy into the process and make the changes necessary to succeed, so the odds that you will do so the second time around with a surgery that probably won't give you as many tools to use are very low. In other words, if you didn't figure out a different coping mechanism the first time around, you probably won't do it the second time either.

Bottom line? You should treat your weight loss surgery as your last chance to get healthy, because it probably is.

The war is never really over. You'll fight it until you die, hopefully at a very old age of natural causes. But, when you're at a healthy weight, you're now fighting the same war as everyone else. Despite what starlets say in the celebrity magazines, there are very few genetic freaks who don't have to watch what they eat and never exercise, yet miraculously stay thin. You're now in the same army fighting against the same enemy as the rest of the population.

You're in a war you can win.

CHAPTER FOURTEEN

War Manual: All You Really Need to Know

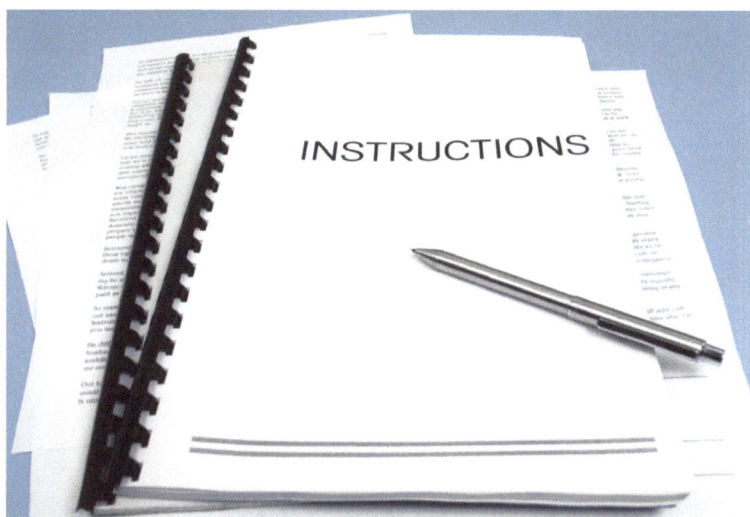

1. The day you decide not to get weight loss surgery is the best you're ever going to feel. It's downhill from there.

2. The day you decide to get weight loss surgery is the worst you'll ever feel. It gets better from there.

3. Running away from your enemy ultimately takes more energy than facing it.

4. If you're a dieting failure, you're in the super majority. Ninety-eight percent of people have also failed.

5. Of the 98% who failed at traditional dieting, 60 to 75% (depending on the procedure) succeeded at losing weight <u>and maintaining it</u> with weight loss surgery.

6. Massive change always involves fear. No one decides to drastically change their life unless something propels them to do so, and that something usually involves tears and anxiety.

7. Your only real enemy is yourself, and that's an enemy you can control given the proper help.

8. You can do this.

www.ingramcontent.com/pod-product-compliance
Lightning Source LLC
Chambersburg PA
CBHW040127270326
41927CB00001B/12